ESSENTIALS OF ANESTHESIOLOGY

SECOND EDITION

DAVID C. CHUNG, M.D.

Consultant Anaesthetist
The Mississauga Hospital
Mississauga, Ontario, Canada

ARTHUR M. LAM, M.D.

Associate Professor, Department of Anesthesiology
University of Washington
Seattle, Washington

Foreword by **Thomas F. Hornbein, M.D.**

Professor and Chairman, Department of Anesthesiology
University of Washington School of Medicine
Seattle, Washington

W. B. SAUNDERS COI
A Division of Harcourt Brace &

Philadelphia, London, Toronto, Montreal, Sydney, Tokyo

W. B. SAUNDERS COMPANY
A Division of
Harcourt Brace & Company

The Curtis Center
Independence Square West
Philadelphia, PA 19106

Library of Congress Cataloging-in-Publication Data

Chung, David C.
    Essentials of anesthesiology.
    Includes index.
    1. Anesthesiology—Handbooks, manuals, etc.   I. Lam, Arthur M.   II. Title.
[DNLM: 1. Anesthesia.
WO 200 C559e]
RD82.2.C48   1990   617.9'6   89-6401
ISBN 0-7216-3084-7

Acquisition Editor: Richard Zorab

Essentials of Anesthesiology   ISBN 0-7216-3084-7

Last digit is the print number: 9   8   7   6   5   4

Foreword

My first teachings as a fledgling anesthesiologist were to drip ether onto a gauze-covered mask skillfully enough to effect a smooth induction without drowning my patient with pungent anesthetic. Monitoring consisted of a finger on the pulse, a blood pressure cuff, and the information provided by closely observing the patient; for example, movement of the chest and abdomen allowed one to assess the depth of anesthesia. At that time role models were few, and as I entered my chosen specialty I wondered what it would be like and whether I had made the right choice.

Now, a third of a century later, I reflect upon the evolution of anesthesiology and upon my good fortune to have been able to grow up with it. Abetted by technological advances unimagined when I began, blood gas measurements, the ability to assess on a moment-to-moment basis such things as intravascular pressures and flows, the practice of critical care medicine has been superimposed upon our earlier knowledge, skills, and art. We are learning to provide safe passage for older, sicker, more fragile patients through more complex, stressful, and prolonged surgical procedures. We have acquired a sophisticated knowledge of physiology and pathophysiology and the ability to titrate an impressive pharmacopeia of potent medications. We still have much to learn in the application of this knowledge and technology to improve outcome, but we are making progress.

However, the foundation upon which this evolution of anesthesiology has taken place is still quite recognizable. Among the joys of being an anesthesiologist is the satisfaction of performing skills with virtuosity, whether in the smooth transition past stage II to surgical sleep with open drop ether or the dexterous placement of an endotracheal tube, epidural needle, or Swan-Ganz catheter; the skill of talking a young child to sleep with neither of you screaming; or the awakening of a patient immediately after surgery with a smile of appreciation on his or her face.

One of my fears when I began was that patients would be mostly asleep and communication would be lacking. I have been delighted to discover another reward, namely the capacity to help a frightened fellow human being through a time of uncertainty, of surrendering control of one's own destiny into the hands of another person. I take pride in the Valium-equivalents, which can be provided by attentive, caring preoperative communication.

This book is a clear and concise introduction to that all-important foundation of anesthesia upon which clinical skill and advanced knowledge can build. It will serve as an excellent basic text for medical students and nurses. Beginning residents should also find it useful. Anesthesia is a risky business. Too much of anesthesia's mortality and morbidity still occurs in healthy patients undergoing simple surgery: preventable mishaps resulting from human or machine failure or sometimes from happenings that we do not yet understand. This book by Drs. Chung and Lam focuses on the fundamental and, in a way, most precious part of what anesthesiology is all about.

Thomas F. Hornbein, M.D.

Acknowledgments

All our students and colleagues have devoted ideas and time to the completion of this edition. Many pharmaceutical companies and equipment manufacturers also have shared technical and research data on their products with us. We are especially indebted to the following: Mrs. Tsai-O Wong, Librarian, the Mississauga Hospital, Mississauga, Canada; Dr. Imelda Bourke, Specialist Anaesthetist, Princess Alexandra Hospital, Brisbane, Australia; Shawn Shaffer, secretary; Trudi Peek, medical illustrator; and Ed Kohnstamm, photographer, all of Harborview Medical Center, University of Washington, Seattle, Washington; Burroughs Wellcome Incorporated; Janssen Pharmaceutica Incorporated; North American Dräger; Ohmeda, The BOC Group Incorporated; and Organon Canada Limited.

Preface
to the First Edition

Anesthesia is a recognized subject in the curriculum of most medical teaching facilities, and many monographs have been published on the subject. However, we have had difficulty in recommending a basic textbook for our students. Indeed, there is more than one good introductory anesthesiology textbook on the market, but they are directed more to students at an intermediate level rather than to those being introduced to the specialty for the first time. The idea of writing this book was conceived to fill this need, and our students and colleagues urged us on.

Anesthetic procedures can be learned only in the operating room. The goal of this book is to provide the scientific basis of anesthesia, not to replace practical experience. In twenty-four chapters, anesthesia-related problems in the patient undergoing surgery are defined and the principles of safe anesthetic practice are discussed. Every attempt to be comprehensive and concise has been made so that the reader can easily acquire a firm foundation in anesthesiology. The student is encouraged to regard this book as his companion—to bring it with him to the ward and into the operating room; to read it; and to refer to it.

Anesthesiology is still a growing specialty. Many of our colleagues are practicing only in areas of special interest in the operating room—for example, in cardiovascular and thoracic surgery or neurosurgery; others are active in the emergency room, the intensive care unit, and the pain clinic. We have chosen to limit the scope of this book to the principles of surgical anesthesia and resuscitation. Other than the anesthetic management of obstetric, pediatric, geriatric, and ambulatory patients, areas of subspecialty are omitted by intention; we feel that the student should not be expected to be involved in these areas in an introductory course.

Although this book is written for clinical clerks, it should be a useful primer for all students of anesthesia. It should also be instructive for physicians, dental surgeons, nurses, and respiratory technicians who are involved in the care of the surgical patient. We trust this book will serve the needs of many, and we welcome the opinion of our readers.

DAVID C. CHUNG

ARTHUR M. LAM

Preface
to the Second Edition

When preparing this new edition, we were troubled with what should reasonably be included in an introductory textbook of anesthesiology. After all, the specialty has made progress in many areas: monitoring, new drugs, management of surgical pain, definition of standards of safe practice, quality assurance, and so forth. In the end we have included all these topics and revised others, but have increased the length of the text only slightly. We believe this edition retains the basic conciseness and comprehensiveness of the first edition. We trust it will continue to serve as a companion to our students; and again we welcome the opinion of our readers.

DAVID C. CHUNG

ARTHUR M. LAM

Contents

General Anesthesia—
Basic Principles

On the tombstone of William T. G. Morton (1819–1868), a pioneer anesthetist, the inscription reads:

Inventor and Revealer of Inhalation Anesthesia;
Before Whom, in All Times, Surgery was Agony;
By Whom, Pain in Surgery was Averted and Annulled;
Since Whom, Science has Control of Pain.

William Morton was a dentist credited with the public demonstration of ether anesthesia on October 16, 1846 at the Massachusetts General Hospital in Boston, nearly 2 years after Horace Wells, another dentist, had failed to convince his surgical colleagues at the same hospital of the anesthetic property of nitrous oxide. Within weeks, ether anesthesia was practiced across the United States and Canada and was received with equal enthusiasm in Great Britain and continental Europe. The following year James Simpson, a Scottish obstetrician, introduced chloroform as an alternative to ether, and in 1863 Gardner Q. Colton re-established nitrous oxide as an adjunct in anesthesia practice. During these early years of inhalation anesthesia, morphine quickly established itself as a preanesthetic medication and as an intraoperative supplement.

The dawn of intravenous anesthesia came in 1873 when Pierre-Cyprien Ore of Bordeaux published his experience with intravenous chloral; but this technique was not firmly established until 1935 when J. S. Lundy of the Mayo Clinic demonstrated the safe use of thiopental, which is still the most popular induction agent in use today. Although the muscle relaxant curare has been used to treat spastic disorders for a number of years, it was not until 1942 that Harold Griffith, of Montreal, reported its use in surgical anesthesia. The discovery of the four groups of anesthetic drugs used in modern practice (intravenous anesthetics, inhalation agents, narcotic analgesics, and muscle relaxants) spanned 100 years. Since then new agents have been introduced in each group to meet specific needs. At the same time, the science and practice of anesthesia has developed into a well-recognized medical specialty called anesthesiology. No longer is the anesthesiologist only an averter and annuller of surgical pain. The anesthesiologist works hand in hand with the surgeon and other medical colleagues to evaluate and prepare patients before surgery, is the patient's primary-care physician during the intraoperative period, and has direct input into the postoperative management of the patient. Using expertise gained in the operating room, the anesthesiologist has also become a significant contributor in other areas of health care, such as the intensive care unit and the pain clinic.

In English-speaking countries other than the United States, the anesthesiologist is commonly called an "anesthetist." This term, although perhaps confusing to American students, is entirely reasonable, as one who administers an anesthetic is an anesthetist. In the United States, only half the anesthetics given annually are administered by anesthesiologists (physician anesthetists); the other half are given by nurse anesthetists. Whereas the anesthesiologist is a graduate physician who has spent 4 years or more of postgraduate training in the management of surgical patients (inside and outside the operating suite), of critically ill patients in intensive care and trauma units, and of patients with acute or chronic pain syndromes, the certified registered nurse anesthetist (CRNA) is a professional who has had 2 years of postgraduate training in surgical anesthesia after basic nursing education. In many hospitals and clinics, nurse anesthetists are integral members of the surgical team.

MOLECULAR MECHANISMS OF ANESTHETIC ACTION

Anesthesia can be defined as a state of reversible loss of sensation and consciousness. A large number of agents, ranging from inert gases to organic compounds, can induce the general anesthetic state. The diversity of molecular species that can produce this state and the lack of a structure-activity relationship have eliminated drug-receptor interaction as a possible mechanism of action.

At the turn of the century, Meyer and Overton observed a direct relationship between potency of inhalation anesthetics and their solubility in oil. More recently it has been confirmed that the minimum alveolar concentration required to maintain anesthesia is lower for more lipid-soluble inhalation agents and higher for less-soluble ones (see "Minimum Alveolar Concentration," Chap. 3). The Meyer-Overton rule implies that inhalation anesthetics act on the lipid environ of the brain, and neuronal membranes of phospholipids have been suggested as the site of action. In addition to lipid solubility, other physicochemical properties and biological activities of anesthetic drugs have been related to their action. Nevertheless, a unified theory of anesthesia remains to be formulated. Some of the classic hypotheses are summarized below.

Lipid Solubility Hypothesis.   There is more than one version of this hypothesis relating lipid solubility to action. The *volume expansion hypothesis* postulates that anesthetic drug molecules taken into the lipid matrix of neuronal membrane cause expansion of these sites and increase lateral pressure on ionic channels penetrating the membrane. When a critical degree of expansion is reached, ion flux through these channels is obstructed and neuronal excitability is inhibited. The *membrane fluidization hypothesis,* on the other hand, proposes that ionic channels are embedded in a bimolecular layer of phospholipids arranged orderly in the gel phase. The presence of anesthetic drugs increases the motility and disrupts the orderly arrangement of these lipid molecules: i.e., a transition from gel to fluid phase has occurred. As a result, the ionic channels lose their structural support and function. In a more elaborate version of the fluidization hypothesis, it is said that closed ionic channels in axonal membrane are surrounded immediately by phospholipids in the fluid phase and by those in gel phase farther lateral (Fig. 1–1A). During excitation the channels spring open for passage of ions—a process facilitated by transforming some of the lipids from high-volume fluid phase to low-volume gel phase (Fig. 1–1B). In the presence of anesthetic molecules, some of the outlying gel-phase lipids become more fluid (Fig. 1–1C), and these fluid-phase lipids fail to condense into the low-volume gel phase, so there will not be room for the ion channels to open on receiving a stimulus (Fig. 1–1D). Consequently the channels become obstructed and neuronal excitation is inhibited.

Protein Interaction Hypothesis.   Although the neuronal membrane is largely a bimolecular layer of phospholipids, ion channels reside in globular proteins penetrating the full thickness of the membrane. The protein interaction hypothesis postulates that molecules of anesthetic bound to hydrophobic sites on these proteins cause the proteins to unfold, which in turn interferes with ion flux–associated neural transmission.

Hydrate Crystal Hypothesis.   Despite the Meyer-Overton rule, not all investigators regard lipid neuronal membrane as the only possible site of anesthetic action. It is known that intermolecular forces can align water molecules around anesthetic molecules to form hydrate or clathrate crystals (structures similar to the orderly arrangement of water molecules in ice crystals). One version suggests that the formation of these microcrystals in the aqueous environ of the brain entraps "ions and electrically charged side chains of protein molecules in such a way as to decrease the energy

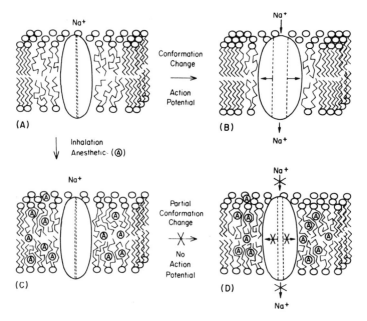

FIGURE 1–1. Diagrammatic illustration of lateral phase separations, a version of the lipid solubility hypothesis of the action of gaseous anesthetics. (From Trudell JR: A unitary theory of anesthesia based on lateral phase separations in nerve membrane. Anesthesiology 46:5–10, 1977. Reproduced with permission of the publisher.)

of electric oscillations in the brain," thus causing loss of consciousness. Another proposes that these crystals plug up the pores of neuronal membranes, raise the threshold of nerve conduction, and affect the binding, hydrolysis, and diffusion of neurotransmitters.

Microtubular Depolymerization Hypothesis. Microtubules are tubular structures made up of protein subunits joined longitudinally. Their abundance in mammalian nerve cells may be related to axonal and synaptic transmission. The observation that halothane can cause reversible disappearance of microtubules from nerve axons suggests that the breakdown or depolymerization of these structures into their protein subunits may be related to the phenomenon of narcosis. However, the ability of halothane and other anesthetics to depolymerize neuronal microtubules has been challenged.

NEUROPHYSIOLOGIC MECHANISMS OF ANESTHETIC ACTION

There is no consensus on the mechanism of action of anesthetic drugs on nerve cells or neuronal pathways. Depression of impulse conduction, synaptic transmission, and activities of specific neuronal units, as well as interaction with opioid receptors, are areas under investigation.

Impulse Conduction. Volatile anesthetics and alcohols interrupt impulse conduction only at concentrations above the clinical range. However, it is speculated that even partial conduction blockade, by decreasing the amount of neurotransmitter released with each impulse, can interfere with synaptic transmission.

Synaptic Transmission. The process of synaptic transmission involves release of a chemical transmitter by the presynaptic neuron, the interaction of transmitter molecules with specific receptors on the postsynaptic membrane, and depolarization of the postsynaptic membrane. There is no evidence to suggest that anesthetic drugs cause depletion of neural transmitters in presynaptic neurons, and the effect of anesthetics on transmitter release is unclear. Owing to the lack of a structure-activity relationship, anesthetic drugs do not act as competitive antagonists at postsynaptic receptor sites, but there is ample proof that inhalation anesthetics depress postsynaptic depolarization at excitatory synapses, and to a much lesser degree at inhibitory synapses.

Specific Neuronal Units. Since the reticular formation is responsible for "arousal," it is tempting to relate the phenomenon of anesthesia to depression of reticular formation activity. Indeed earlier experiments were confirmatory; however, there is evidence that cortical neurons and long tracts of the spinal cord are as sensitive as the reticular formation to the action of anesthetic drugs. The current view is that anesthetics can act on multiple sites rather than on a single region of the central nervous system; monosynaptic and multisynaptic units are equally sensitive.

Opioid Receptors. The fact that naloxone, a pure narcotic antagonist, reverses some of the effects of volatile anesthetics has led to the speculation that these drugs produce narcosis through interaction with the opioid receptor–endorphin system. The exact mode of interaction is as yet unclear.

STAGES OF ETHER ANESTHESIA

Although the mode of action of anesthetic drugs is not fully understood, their clinical effects can be described accurately. Guedel described the progressive depression of the central nervous system by ether in four stages—analgesia, excitement, surgical anesthesia, and impending death.

Analgesia (Stage I).   The stage of analgesia lasts from onset of drowsiness to loss of eyelash reflex (blinking in response to stroking of the eyelash).

Excitement (Stage II).   The stage of excitement is characterized by agitation and delirium. Respiration is irregular, and copious salivation can occur. Pupils are large, and the eyes are divergent. Toward the end of this stage, respiration is again rhythmic (automatic respiration).

Surgical Anesthesia (Stage III).   This stage is subdivided into four planes:

Plane 1   In this plane respiration is rhythmic, and rapid side-to-side eye movement is seen.

Plane 2   This plane lasts from cessation of rapid eye movement to onset of paresis of intercostal muscles.

Plane 3   This plane lasts from onset of paresis of intercostal muscles to paralysis of these muscles.

Plane 4   This plane lasts from paralysis of intercostal muscles to paralysis of the diaphragm. The patient ceases to breathe at the end of this plane.

Impending Death (Stage IV).   The stage of impending death lasts from onset of apnea to failure of the circulation and represents medullary depression.

COMPONENTS OF GENERAL ANESTHESIA

With replacement of ether by nonflammable agents and with the advent of intravenous drugs and muscle relaxants, the stages and signs of ether anesthesia are no longer observed. Instead, G. J. Rees and T. C. Gray described the state of general anesthesia in terms of three basic components: the triad of unconsciousness (hypnosis), analgesia (areflexia), and muscle relaxation.

Unconsciousness (Hypnosis).   With development of unconsciousness, the patient is oblivious to all sensation, but somatic and autonomic reflexes to pain and noxious stimuli can still occur.

Analgesia (Areflexia).   Withdrawal of a limb or flight (somatic reflexes) and hypertension, tachycardia, and sweating (autonomic reflexes) are part of the subconscious reaction to pain. These potent reflexes must be subdued during anesthesia.

Muscle Relaxation.   The degree of muscle relaxation required varies according to the operation. In general, only a mild degree of muscle relaxation is necessary for superficial operations on body wall or extremities, but moderate to profound muscle relaxation is required for operations within body cavities.

ANESTHETIC DRUGS

In the past, the triad of general anesthesia was obtained by progressive depression of the central nervous system with ether or chloroform alone. In current practice, a multiplicity of agents with specific actions are used to provide unconsciousness, analgesia, and muscle relaxation. These include intravenous anesthetics (used mainly for induction of anesthesia), inhalation anesthetics (used for maintenance of unconsciousness), narcotic analgesics, and muscle relaxants. The pharmacology of these agents is discussed in Chapters 2 through 5.

Intravenous Anesthetics

The intravenous route is a popular method for administration of drugs used in anesthetic practice. Injection of a drug directly into the circulation allows rapid distribution to the site of action with generally quick onset of action. By giving the drug in small increments, dose can be titrated against effects. Once the desired effects are achieved, they can be maintained by continuous infusion.

The intravenous route is not without drawbacks. Once the drug is injected, its effect cannot be reversed readily and there is potential for catastrophe. Side-effects can be unexpectedly severe as a result of the high, though transient, plasma concentration attained following rapid intravenous injection, and the danger of anaphylaxis is ever present. In addition, phlebitis and thrombophlebitis are relatively common problems. Unless sterile technique is followed, the intravenous route can become the gateway for bacteria, pyrogens, and other foreign bodies to enter the circulation. Last but not least, there is the risk of fluid overload in some patients (e.g., small infants).

PHARMACOKINETICS

When plasma concentration of an intravenous anesthetic (e.g., thiopental) is plotted on a logarithmic scale against time after it is given intravenously as a bolus, the curve thus obtained has three distinct features (Fig. 2–1). An initial peak is followed by a phase of rapid decline in plasma level (the distribution phase) and a later phase of slower decline (the elimination phase).

Peak Concentration

Following a bolus injection, plasma concentration peaks within one or two circulations of the drug in the body. The drug-laden blood circulates most rapidly to the vessel-rich group of organs, where the drug is taken up instantaneously (see "Tissue Blood Flow and Tissue Mass," below). This period of peak plasma con-

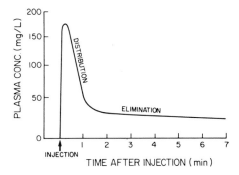

FIGURE 2–1.   The rise and fall in plasma concentration of an intravenous anesthetic following injection of a bolus.

centration is only transient. As tissue uptake progresses, plasma concentration falls.

Distribution

The initial phase of relatively rapid decline in plasma level is known as the *distribution phase (α-phase)*. During this period, decline in plasma level is almost solely the result of distribution and redistribution of drug to and uptake of drug by various organs. Pharmacologic effect of intravenous anesthetics is determined by drug concentration in brain tissue, which is largely related to blood level. Therefore, the rate at which plasma level falls determines the duration of action after a single bolus injection of intravenous anesthetic. The rate of this decline (i.e., the slope of the distribution phase) is determined by tissue uptake. Several factors act independently to influence tissue uptake and therefore this decline: protein binding, physical characteristics of the drug, and tissue blood flow and tissue mass.

Protein Binding

In the circulation, all intravenous anesthetics are bound to plasma protein (usually albumin), but the degree of binding varies according to the agent used. Since only free non-protein-bound drugs can diffuse across cell membranes, protein binding decreases tissue uptake and slows the decline in plasma level during the distribution phase. These binding sites are nonspecific, so many foreign compounds can compete for them. In the presence of such a substance or in the event of a decreased plasma concentration of albumin (e.g., in liver disease), more of the drug will be present in the unbound form after intravenous injection of a usual dose. Since unbound drugs are pharmacologically active, this higher concentration of free drug can be the cause of an unexpected overdose.

Physical Characteristics of the Drug

Some physical characteristics of the drug itself are major determinants of how rapidly it is taken up by tissues. These include lipid solubility, molecular size, and the state of ionization.

Of these, *lipid solubility* is the most important. Highly lipid-soluble drugs (e.g., all intravenous anesthetics) are taken up rapidly by tissues. Lipid-soluble drugs also pass readily into "special circulations" (e.g., brain and placenta).

With water-soluble agents, *molecular size* is an important determinant of diffusibility across plasma membranes. The smaller the molecule, the more easily it can cross into tissue. With highly lipid-souble agents, molecular weight plays little role in influencing diffusibility.

For drugs that are ionizable, the *state of ionization* greatly affects how rapidly they enter tissues. Only nonionized molecules diffuse across membranes readily. An equilibrium exists across plasma membranes only for the nonionized form of a drug, so the total drug concentration (the ionized plus the nonionized fractions) on either side of the membrane can be very different. The pK_a of a drug is the pH at which 50% of the drug is ionized. The degree of ionization is determined by this value and the ambient pH, according to the Henderson-Hasselbalch equation:

$$pK_a - pH = \log\frac{[\text{acid form of drug}]}{[\text{base form of drug}]}$$

This equation can be rearranged for convenience as follows:

$$\frac{[\text{acid form of drug}]}{[\text{base form of drug}]} = \text{antilog } (pK_a - pH)$$

There is more acid form than base form of the drug when the difference between pK_a and pH is positive; there is more base form when the difference is negative. A drug is an acid if it is a donor of protons; it is a base if it is an acceptor of protons. Depending on the particular drug, the ionized fraction can be either a base or an acid. For example, the ionized fraction of sodium thiopental (NaTP) is a base. It can accept a proton according to the formulas:

$$\underset{\text{sodium salt}}{\text{NaTP}} \rightleftharpoons Na^+ + \underset{\text{ionized base}}{TP^-}$$

$$\underset{\text{ionized base}}{TP^-} + \underset{\text{proton}}{H^+} \rightleftharpoons \underset{\text{nonionized acid}}{HTP}$$

On the other hand, the ionized fraction of lidocaine hydrochloride (XHCl) is an acid. It can donate a proton according to the formulas:

$$\underset{\text{hydrochloride salt}}{XHCl} \quad \rightleftharpoons \quad \underset{\text{ionized acid}}{XH^+} \quad + \quad Cl^-$$

$$\underset{\text{ionized acid}}{XH^+} \quad \rightleftharpoons \quad \underset{\text{nonionized base}}{X} \quad + \quad \underset{\text{proton}}{H^+}$$

Ion trapping is a phenomenon related to this pH-dependent ionization of many molecules when there is a pH difference across cell membranes. It is the cause of increase in urinary excretion of salicylate with alkalinization of urine. Sodium salicylate (NaS) can exist as an ionized base or a nonionized acid, according to the formulas:

$$\underset{\text{sodium salt}}{NaS} \quad \rightleftharpoons Na^+ + \quad \underset{\text{ionized base}}{S^-}$$

$$\underset{\text{ionized base}}{S^-} \quad + \quad \underset{\text{proton}}{H^+} \rightleftharpoons \quad \underset{\text{nonionized acid}}{HS}$$

After the nonionized acid has crossed into the lumen of renal tubules, a highly alkaline urine (i.e., urine abundant in hydroxyl ions) favors the equilibrium heavily to the right of the equation:

$$\underset{\text{nonionized acid}}{HS} \quad + \quad \underset{\text{hydroxyl ion}}{OH^-} \quad \rightleftharpoons \quad \underset{\text{ionized base}}{S^-} \quad + \quad H_2O$$

Therefore most of the salicylate will exist as negatively charged ions "trapped" in the tubular lumen. They cannot be reabsorbed from the urine and are excreted.

Tissue Blood Flow and Tissue Mass

All intravenous anesthetics are highly soluble in lipid; they are taken up readily by most tissues. The major factors influencing tissue uptake are tissue blood flow and tissue mass.

The tissues of the body can be divided into four groups according to their regional blood flow. Approximately 70% of the cardiac output goes to vessel-rich viscera (brain, heart, liver, kidneys), 25% to lean body mass (muscle), 4% to fat, and only 1% to the vessel-poor group (skin, cartilage, bone). Following bolus injection, a drug is first distributed to tissues receiving the greatest portion of cardiac output. Distribution to the vessel-poor group usually can be ignored.

Distribution of thiopental among the plasma pool and other tissues after a single injection is illustrated in Figure 2–2. As the fraction in the plasma pool falls, it is first taken up by the brain and other visceral organs, which account for only a tenth of body

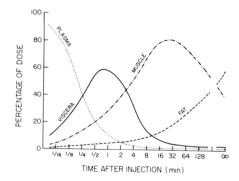

FIGURE 2–2. The distribution and redistribution of thiopental among the plasma pool, viscera, muscle, and fat following the intravenous injection of a bolus. (From Price HL, Linde HW, Price ML: Clin Pharmacol Ther 1:298, 1960.)

weight. The fraction taken up by this vessel-rich group of tissues peaks at 30 seconds to 1 minute after injection. As time goes on, the fraction taken up by skeletal muscle, which accounts for approximately half of total body weight and has a relatively good blood supply, becomes more significant. This fraction surpasses that in the viscera by 5 minutes and peaks at approximately 20 minutes, while the fraction accumulated in brain and viscera falls. It is this redistribution of thiopental from brain to lean body mass that accounts for emergence from anesthesia after a single injection of this agent. Fat accounts for nearly a fifth of body weight and has a high affinity for fat-soluble agents, but its blood supply is relatively poor. For this reason, the fraction of thiopental taken up by fat becomes significant only at a much later point in time. This accumulation of thiopental in fat and its slow elimination are responsible for its residual sedative effect.

Elimination

The phase of slower decline in plasma level represented by the latter portion of the graph in Figure 2–1 is the *elimination phase* (β-*phase*). It is mainly the result of effective elimination of the intravenous anesthetic from the body. Elimination by metabolism and by excretion of the drug and its metabolites in bile or urine gains importance in governing recovery following repeated injections or continuous infusion of an intravenous anesthetic. It starts almost immediately after injection, but its contribution to the decline in plasma level during the distribution phase is masked by rapid tissue uptake. Only after the distribution phase has almost run its course does the elimination phase become evident. Likewise, distribution and redistribution continue at a slow pace during the phase of elimination.

Metabolism

With few exceptions, intravenous anesthetics are broken down by mixed-function oxidases, also known as the cytochrome P450 system, closely associated with the endoplasmic reticulum in liver cells. The enzymatic activity of this system is normally relatively low, but it can be increased several-fold by pretreatment with many substances foreign to the body, a phenomenon known as enzyme induction.

Most intravenous anesthetics are metabolized along oxidative pathways. These usually involve hydroxylation, but sometimes also dealkylation, deamination, demethylation, and desulfuration. Frequently the drug and its metabolites are conjugated with glucuronic acid and rendered water-soluble before excretion.

Excretion

Excretion of intravenous anesthetics and their metabolites from the body occurs mainly in the kidneys. Renal excretion involves both glomerular filtration of the non-protein-bound fraction and tubular secretion of both the bound and unbound fractions. After excretion, drugs may be reabsorbed in the tubules to a varying degree. This tubular reabsorption is dependent upon the same physical characteristics discussed earlier: lipid solubility enhances reabsorption and delays excretion, whereas ionization impedes reabsorption and enhances excretion. Occasionally, specific transport mechanisms are involved in reabsorption.

Intravenous anesthetics also may be excreted via the biliary tract after being metabolized and conjugated in the liver. In general this route is less important than that via the kidneys, but it can assume much greater importance in renal failure.

SPECIFIC AGENTS

Intravenous anesthetics have a rapid onset and short duration of action. They are commonly given in a bolus for induction of anesthesia. Occasionally they are given repeatedly or infused slowly to maintain anesthesia.

Thiopental

Thiopental, the most commonly used induction agent in modern clinical practice, is a derivative of barbituric acid. It is an ultra-short-acting barbiturate, and its anesthetic action is obvious within one arm-to-brain circulation time. Induction of anesthesia with thiopental is pleasant. The induction dose is 3–5 mg/kg, which should be given slowly (over 30–60 seconds) during induction, so that the dose can be titrated against observed effects.

Thiopental has a pK_a of 7.6. Almost 60% of the molecules are in the nonionized form at normal body pH. In the presence of acidemia, even less is ionized. This drug is also highly soluble in lipids, and approximately 70% of an injected dose is protein bound. Decrease in plasma protein concentration (e.g., in patients with hepatic disease) or presence of substances competing for binding sites on these protein molecules may result in overdose following the administration of a usual clinical dose.

The duration of anesthetic action following an induction dose is approximately 5 minutes. This ultrashort action is a result of rapid redistribution of the drug from brain to muscle. It is broken down in the liver by oxidation and conjugation. Normally detoxification occurs at a rate of 10–15% per hour, and less than 1% of an injected dose is excreted unchanged in urine. This slow rate of elimination is responsible for the residual sedative effect seen with thiopental during recovery.

Thiopental for injection is prepared as a 2.5% solution of the sodium salt, which has a pH of 10.8. While extravascular injection of such an alkaline solution can produce tissue necrosis, intra-arterial injection will cause severe arterial spasm that may result in ischemic necrosis of tissues supplied by the artery. Therefore sodium thiopental should be given only via a secure and freely running intravenous line.

The effect of thiopental on the central nervous system is complex. Following induction of anesthesia, there is a fall in cerebral oxygen demand accompanied by a similar fall in cerebral blood flow. Intracranial pressure also declines. On this basis it has been suggested that thiopental may protect the brain from hypoxic or ischemic insults. This principle forms the basis for the induction of barbiturate coma in patients with cerebrovascular accidents and head injuries. Recent evidence suggests that it is not useful in global hypoxia or ischemia but can offer protection when given before the occurrence of focal ischemic events. A reduction in postoperative neurologic dysfunction following cardiopulmonary bypass for valve surgery also has been reported.

Thiopental has no analgesic properties. In fact, it is said to be antianalgesic because it appears to increase the subjective feeling of pain at subanesthetic doses. It depresses the vasomotor center of the brain stem, depresses the myocardium, and encourages peripheral vascular pooling, all of which can combine to produce hypotension. It must be given with extreme caution to patients with hypovolemia or myocardial disease. Since thiopental also depresses the respiratory center at the brain stem, transient apnea following a normal induction dose is not unusual. Thiopental is contraindicated when a patient's airway or ventilation cannot be guaranteed following induction of anesthesia.

Injection of thiopental into a vein can produce wheals and flares along the course of the vein as well as a characteristic mottled erythematous flush over the upper chest and neck. Both phenomena are related to the release of histamine. An increased incidence of bronchospasm in asthmatics following administration of thiopental is also attributed to this histamine-releasing property. It is absolutely contraindicated in patients acutely ill with asthma, and it is relatively contraindicated in those whose disease is in remission.

Like other barbiturates, thiopental can precipitate an acute crisis in patients who have porphyria and, so, is contraindicated for them. Other contraindications include hypothyroidism and a history of hypersensitivity to other barbiturates.

Thiamylal

Like thiopental, thiamylal is also a thiobarbiturate. These two compounds are comparable in potency and action.

Methohexital

Methohexital is another ultrashort-acting barbiturate frequently used for the induction of anesthesia. Unlike thiopental, methohexital is an oxybarbiturate. The induction dose is approximately 1–2 mg/kg.

Methohexital has two major advantages over thiopental: an earlier recovery time and less cumulative effect with repeated injections; however induction of anesthesia with methohexital is associated with a higher incidence of excitatory phenomena (cough, hiccup, and other involuntary movements). It is also associated with a transient but unpleasant ache at the site of injection.

Diazepam

Diazepam, a benzodiazepine, is a minor tranquilizer that has found widespread use in anesthesia practice: for preanesthesia sedation, for sedation during local anesthesia, and occasionally for induction of general anesthesia. It is noted for its lack of cardiovascular side-effects, even at high doses, but it can cause mild respiratory depression. It is also an effective anticonvulsant and has a mild relaxant effect on skeletal muscles. The latter action is probably a result of inhibition of spinal reflexes.

When diazepam is used to induce general anesthesia, the onset of action is gradual (2–5 minutes), and a wide variation in dose requirement is observed (0.15–1.5 mg/kg). Therefore the dose should be titrated against the desired effect. Since it is highly lipid soluble, a large fraction of diazepam is stored in body fat following intravenous administration. Ultimately it is metabolized in the liver, but its metabolites are only slightly less active than the parent compound and are responsible for its prolonged sedative action following administration of a large bolus. Consequently diazepam is used only occasionally for induction of anesthesia. Over 70% of its metabolites are excreted in urine, and approximately 10% in feces.

Valium is injectable diazepam prepared in an organic solvent of mixed composition (40% propylene glycol, 10% ethyl alcohol, 5% sodium benzoate and benzoic acid, 1.5% benzyl alcohol). It becomes cloudy when mixed with aqueous intravenous solutions, but there is no apparent loss of potency. Pain at the site of injection is common when it is given intravenously, and the incidence of phlebitis is high. *Diazemuls* is an injectable emulsion of diazepam prepared in fractionated soybean oil, acetylated monoglycerides, fractionated egg phospholipids, and glycerol with sodium hydroxide added to adjust the pH to 8. This latter preparation is said to be less irritating to tissues.

Midazolam

Midazolam, a water-soluble benzodiazepine, has all the pharmacologic actions of diazepam and is associated with a higher frequency of anterograde amnesia. It is two to three times more potent than diazepam, causes little venous irritation, and can be given intramuscularly. Rapid intravenous injection of midazolam can cause hypotension and dose-related respiratory depression. The induction dose is variable (0.15–0.4 mg/kg) and onset of action, gradual. Although its duration of anesthetic action is less than that of diazepam, it is two to three times as long as that of thiopental. This agent is cleared by the liver and excreted as conjugated metabolites in urine; less than 0.03% of a given dose is excreted unchanged.

The relatively long duration of action of both benzodiazepines (diazepam and midazolam) and their potential to cause neonatal depression are major disadvantages of these compounds. *Flumazenil* (Ro 15–1788), an experimental benzodiazepine antagonist, has been shown in clinical trials to be capable of reversing the central nervous system–depressant effect of both diazepam and midazolam. If proved safe, this specific antagonist could change the practice of intravenous sedation and anesthesia using these agents.

Droperidol

Droperidol, a butyrophenone, is a major tranquilizer. It produces a state of cognitive dissociation and is called a neuroleptic.

It is also a useful antiemetic that acts directly on the chemoreceptor trigger zone in the medulla. Although droperidol itself has no analgesic properties, it is used in neuroleptanalgesia, a technique in which it is combined with a narcotic analgesic (usually fentanyl). This technique has been used to supplement regional anesthesia and to sedate patients during invasive diagnostic procedures. Together with fentanyl, nitrous oxide, and a muscle relaxant, droperidol is also used to induce and maintain neuroleptanesthesia.

Droperidol has several noteworthy adverse side-effects. It has some alpha-blocking properties that can cause hypotension when large doses are given; it can cause an anxious, agitated state (dysphoria) in some patients when it is given alone. Occasionally extrapyramidal dyskinesia and parkinsonian rigidity are seen because droperidol interferes with dopaminergic transmission in the central nervous system.

Ketamine

Ketamine is a derivative of cyclohexanone. It produces a dissociative mental state characterized by catalepsy, sedation, amnesia, and analgesia. In anesthetic doses ketamine produces a seizurelike electroencephalogram (EEG) pattern in humans without producing associated muscle activity.

Ketamine can be given intravenously or intramuscularly. The normal dose is 1–2 mg/kg intravenously over 1 minute or 6.5–13 mg/kg intramuscularly. The duration of action is 5–10 minutes after an intravenous dose and 15–25 minutes after an intramuscular injection. This agent is converted to water-soluble metabolites in the liver, which are then excreted in urine. It has found application in pediatric diagnostic procedures, in burn surgery, and in critically ill patients because of its special anesthetic properties and pharmacologic actions discussed in the next paragraph.

Patients under ketamine anesthesia usually retain the laryngeal reflex and can maintain a patent upper airway without assistance, although aspiration and airway obstruction sometimes occur. These properties make ketamine a safer agent when anesthesia is required under primitive conditions, as at the scene of an accident. The effect of ketamine on the cardiovascular system is stimulatory: a rise in blood pressure of 20–40 mm Hg and an increase in heart rate of 30–40 beats per minute are usual. As a result myocardial work is increased, so ketamine is contraindicated in hypertensive patients and in patients with ischemic heart disease. However it is useful for induction of anesthesia in patients who are hypovolemic when the operation is urgent. Since it is a potent bronchodilator, it is also useful for induction of anesthesia in asthmatic patients.

Ketamine is related to the hallucinogens. Emergence from ketamine anesthesia is frequently associated with bad dreams and dysphoria. Patients should be allowed to recover undisturbed in a quiet, dark area. The administration of 5–10 mg of diazepam intravenously can reduce the incidence of emergence delirium without prolonging recovery.

Etomidate

Etomidate, an imidazole derivative formulated in a solvent containing propylene glycol, has an onset and a duration of action similar to those of thiopental. The induction dose is 0.25–0.3 mg/kg. Like thiopental, it decreases cerebral metabolism, cerebral blood flow, and intracranial pressure; but unlike thiopental, it causes only minor respiratory depression, little change in circulatory function, and no histamine release. Therefore it can be used safely in cardiac and asthmatic patients. However it is associated with a high incidence of pain at the site of injection, myoclonic jerks and hiccups (a facilitatory phenomenon not accompanied by epileptiform EEG patterns), and postoperative nausea and vomiting. Because a single dose of etomidate can suppress adrenocortical function for several hours, prolonged infusion to maintain sedation (e.g., in the intensive care unit) is discouraged, but its use as an induction agent is not contraindicated.

Etomidate is cleared rapidly by the liver, where it is hydrolyzed to yield inactive water-soluble breakdown products. Approximately 75% of a given dose is recoverable from urine as metabolites, and another 15% from feces.

Propofol

Propofol (diisopropylphenol) has pharmacologic actions very similar to those of thiopental, but it is cleared by the liver at a much faster rate. Time from emergence to full recovery (orientation) following an induction dose is more rapid than that of any of the intravenous agents described earlier, so it is gaining popularity as an induction agent in outpatient anesthesia. Its rapid elimination and lack of cumulative effect have also made it ideal for use in a continuous infusion to maintain anesthesia in the so-called total intravenous anesthesia technique.

Since propofol is water insoluble, it is formulated as an aqueous emulsion containing 10% soybean oil, 1.2% egg phosphatide, and 2.3% glycerol. The induction dose is 1.5–3 mg/kg.

Inhalation Anesthetics

The first anesthetics introduced into clinical practice were inhalation agents (nitrous oxide, ether, chloroform). They were used for both induction and maintenance of anesthesia. Since the introduction of thiopental in 1934, however, the use of intravenous agents for induction has largely superseded the use of inhalation agents. Nevertheless induction of anesthesia with inhalation anesthetics is still popular in children and in patients in whom intravenous agents are contraindicated. Unlike that with ether, induction with modern inhalation agents is both pleasant for the patient and rapid in onset. Except for transient agitation and irregularity of breathing, the second stage described for ether anesthesia is seldom obvious.

PHARMACOKINETICS

Administration of a drug via the respiratory tract to act on a distant target organ is unique to the practice of anesthesia. Before reviewing alveolar and tissue uptake of inhalation agents, it is necessary to define concentration, partial pressure, and minimum alveolar concentration (MAC) of these agents. These terms apply to both gases and vapors.

Concentration

The fraction of a gas in a mixture is equal to the volume of that gas divided by the total volume of the mixture, and the concentration of this gas in the mixture is this fraction expressed as a percentage. For example, the concentration of nitrous oxide in a mixture of 7 liters of nitrous oxide and 3 liters of oxygen is 70%; a 10-liter mixture of oxygen, nitrous oxide, and 1% halothane has 100 ml of halothane vapor (not the liquid). Concentration is a convenient way of describing the composition of an anesthetic mixture. However concentration gradient is not the force behind the movement of gas molecules between a gas-liquid or a liquid-liquid interface.

Consider the example in Figure 3–1, in which a gas mixture in compartment *A* is separated by a semipermeable membrane from blood in compartment *B*. If halothane is added to compartment *A* so that its final concentration is 1%, some of the halothane molecules will cross into the blood in compartment *B*. With time, an equilibrium will be established, and the number of molecules crossing from compartment *A* into compartment *B* will equal those crossing from compartment *B* into compartment *A*. That is, the net movement of halothane molecules is zero. The force behind this movement of halothane molecules and the eventual state of equilibrium is partial pressure. If compartment *B* is, in turn, separated by another semipermeable membrane from compartment *C* containing tissue fluid as in Figure 3–2, halothane molecules will also cross into compartment *C* until equilibrium is established. At equilibrium, the partial pressures of halothane in all three compartments are equal.

Partial Pressure

Gas molecules are in constant motion, whether they are in a mixture or in solution. Molecules in a gas mixture are constantly bombarding the walls of their container; those in solution are always leaping into the atmosphere above the liquid they are dissolved in or are crossing the boundary of a liquid-liquid interface. Partial pressure (also called *tension*) may be regarded as a measure of these activities.

By definition, the partial pressure of a component gas in a

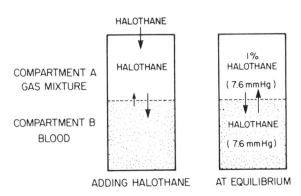

FIGURE 3–1. The movement of halothane across a gas–blood interface. At equilibrium, partial pressures of halothane in both compartments are equal.

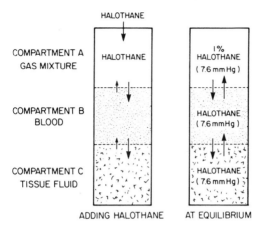

FIGURE 3–2. The movement of halothane across a gas–blood and a blood–tissue fluid interface. At equilibrium, partial pressures in all three compartments are equal.

mixture is equal to the fraction it contributes toward total pressure. That is,

$$\frac{\text{Partial pressure of}}{\text{a component gas}} = \frac{\text{Total pressure}}{\text{of mixture}} \times \frac{\text{Concentration of}}{\text{component gas}}$$

In the example in Figure 3–2, the partial pressure of halothane in compartment *A* is 1% of 760 mm Hg, or 7.6 mm Hg if the total pressure is atmospheric.

When a gas is in solution, its partial pressure can be deduced from the composition of the gas mixture with which the solvent is in equilibrium. At steady state, the partial pressure of the gas in both phases is equal. In the example of Figure 3–2, the partial pressure of halothane in the blood of compartment *B* is equal to that in compartment *A*, 7.6 mm Hg. Similarly, the partial pressure of halothane in the tissue fluid of compartment *C* is 7.6 mm Hg. It should be noted that this example also describes gas exchange between alveolar gas and pulmonary blood, and between blood and tissue fluid.

Minimum Alveolar Concentration

The minimum alveolar concentration, or *MAC*, of an inhalation agent is the concentration of that agent in alveolar gas necessary to prevent movement in 50% of patients when a standard incision is made. Since the MAC is in effect the median effective dose (ED$_{50}$) of an inhalation agent, it follows that an alveolar concentration higher than MAC will be required to retain immobility in the remaining 50% of patients when the same standard stimulus is used. Normally immobility can be achieved in 95% of patients when the alveolar concentration of the anesthetic is 30% above its MAC value.

Alveolar concentration is a convenient method of quantifying the dose of an inhalation agent a patient receives because it can easily be translated into partial pressure. At equilibrium, the partial pressure of the agent in alveolar gas equals that in blood as well as that in the brain (the site of action). The setting of the vaporizer is not a true reflection of the dose received because some of the anesthetic is lost to the rubber of the anesthetic circuit or to the surrounding atmosphere before it reaches the respiratory tract. Nor is the inspired concentration, measured at the upper respiratory tract, an accurate reflection of this dose, because a gradient exists between alveolar and inspired concentrations during the course of a normal anesthetic procedure (see ''Alveolar Uptake,'' below). This dose can be monitored only by measuring end-tidal concentration of the vapor using a halometer, mass spectrometer, or photospectrometer (see Chap. 14).

The MACs of commonly used inhalation agents are listed in Table 3–1. For convenience, the alveolar concentration of an inhalation agent is commonly expressed as a multiple or a fraction of its MAC; for example, an alveolar concentration of 1.54% halothane as 2 MAC of halothane and an alveolar concentration of 0.85% enflurane as 0.5 MAC of enflurane. In general the anesthetic effects and the MACs of inhalation agents used in combination are simply additive. That is, an alveolar concentration of 70% nitrous oxide (0.7 MAC) and an alveolar concentration of 0.57% enflurane (0.3 MAC) will keep 50% of patients immobile when they are subjected to the standard stimulus.

This definition of MAC has made it possible to compare the

TABLE 3–1. MINIMUM ALVEOLAR CONCENTRATION (MAC) OF INHALATION ANESTHETICS

AGENTS (in Order of Decreasing Potency)	MAC (%)
Methoxyflurane	0.16
Halothane	0.77
Isoflurane	1.15
Enflurane	1.7
Nitrous oxide	104

potency of inhalation anesthetics. An agent that has a lower MAC value is more potent than one with a larger MAC value (see Table 3–1). Similarly the definition of MAC allows comparison of side-effects of different agents at equipotent anesthetic doses.

There are many factors that will increase or decrease the MAC of an inhalation agent. Pyrexia and the administration of dextroamphetamine (a drug that promotes the release of catecholamine in the central nervous system) increase MAC. Advancing age, hypothermia, and administration of narcotic analgesics or reserpine (a drug that depletes the central nervous system of catecholamines) all decrease MAC. Other factors that decrease MAC include severe hypercapnia ($PaCO_2 > 90$ mm Hg), severe hypoxemia ($PaO_2 < 40$ mm Hg), and severe anemia (hematocrit $< 10\%$). On the other hand, mild hypercapnia, profound hypocapnia, mild hypoxemia, mild anemia, circadian rhythms, hyperthyroidism, hypothyroidism, and the duration of anesthesia have no discernible effect on MAC.

Alveolar Uptake

As pointed out in the previous section, the alveolar concentration of an inhalation agent must be raised to a certain level in order to achieve anesthesia. At equilibrium, the partial pressure of the anesthetic agent in the alveoli equals that in blood and brain. In practice, the anesthetic is delivered to the upper respiratory tract, from which it is inhaled. The rate of alveolar uptake is gradual and follows an exponential growth pattern illustrated by the curves in Figure 3–3. Equilibration between alveolar concentration and inspired concentration occurs only at infinity and is never reached within the course of an anesthetic procedure.

The rate of alveolar uptake is determined by three different factors—inspired concentration, washout of alveolar gas, and uptake by pulmonary blood. However both washout of alveolar gas and uptake by pulmonary blood are influenced by other independent factors. Those that affect alveolar washout are alveolar ventilation and functional residual capacity, and those that influence uptake by pulmonary blood are solubility of the agent in blood, cardiac output, and alveolar–mixed venous tension gradient.

Inspired Concentration

It is not surprising that the rate of rise in the alveolar concentration of an anesthetic agent is faster if more of it is delivered in the inspired gas mixture. Curve X in Figure 3–3A represents the exponential growth in alveolar concentration of a volatile anesthetic when the inspired concentration is 1%. When inspired concentration is increased to 2%, alveolar concentration will grow along curve Y. The more rapid rate of rise in alveolar concentration

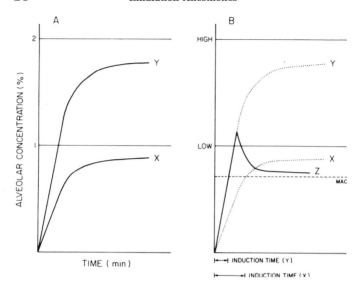

FIGURE 3–3. The influence of inspired concentration on the rate of alveolar uptake and induction time. See text for details.

when inspired concentration is increased is obvious. This effect is seen with both insoluble and soluble agents.

The solution of a soluble agent in blood tends to reduce the rate at which its alveolar concentration increases. The retardant effect on the rate of rise decreases as the inspired concentration increases. This phenomenon is called the *concentration effect*. It is an additional factor that contributes to increasing the rate of alveolar uptake of soluble agents at higher inspired concentrations. The importance of this factor increases with the solubility of the agent. Since all volatile agents currently in use are relatively insoluble, the influence of concentration effect on the alveolar uptake of these agents can be regarded as minimal.

Practical application of this influence of inspired concentration on alveolar uptake is found in inhalation induction. In Figure 3–3B, alveolar uptake follows curve X when a low inspired concentration of inhalation anesthetic is given, but it follows curve Y when the inspired concentration is increased. The consequence of giving a higher inspired concentration during induction is a shorter induction time. Once anesthesia is established, the inspired concentration can be adjusted to lower values for maintenance (curve Z).

Alveolar Ventilation

Because inhalation anesthetics are delivered only to the upper airway, from which they are inhaled, hyperventilation increases the rate of alveolar uptake and hypoventilation decreases it.

Functional Residual Capacity

Functional residual capacity (*FRC*) is the volume of air in the lungs at the end of a normal expiration, which acts as a buffer to changes in the composition of alveolar gas. The time required to complete 63% of alveolar uptake (the *time constant*) is related to FRC and alveolar ventilation per minute ($\dot{V}_A$) by the following formula:

$$\text{Time constant} = \frac{\text{FRC}}{\dot{V}_A}$$

Thus the rate of rise in alveolar concentration is fast (short time constant) when FRC is small or $\dot{V}_A$ large, and the rate of rise is slow (long time constant) when FRC is large or $\dot{V}_A$ small.

Solubility of Anesthetic Agent

The solubility of an inhalation agent in blood is defined as the amount of anesthetic agent required to saturate a unit volume of blood at a given temperature and can be expressed as the blood–gas partition coefficient. The relative solubility of agents in clinical use as expressed by their partition coefficients is as follows:

nitrous oxide < isoflurane < enflurane < halothane < methoxyflurane
  (0.47)   (1.4)   (1.8)   (2.3)   (13.0)

The more soluble is the agent, the greater is the amount that will be carried away by blood in the pulmonary capillaries during uptake. Thus the rate of increase in the alveolar uptake curve is slowed. On the other hand, the alveolar concentration of a relatively insoluble agent increases faster. In practical terms, the solubility of the inhalation agent in blood is the most important single factor in determining the speed of induction and of recovery in individual patients. Induction and recovery are fast with highly insoluble agents and slow with soluble ones.

Cardiac Output

Gases in the alveoli are in equilibrium with blood in the pulmonary capillaries. Therefore how much anesthetic is removed from the lungs by pulmonary blood depends not only on the solubility of the agent but also on pulmonary blood flow. Alveolar anesthetic concentration rises slowly when cardiac output (pulmonary blood flow) is high. Cerebral blood flow usually remains normal in high cardiac output states, and most of the increase in flow is distributed to other tissues. Therefore the slower rise in alveolar anesthetic concentration will slow the induction of anesthesia. Conversely a low cardiac output will allow a faster rise in alveolar concentration and will speed up induction, provided cerebral blood flow is maintained.

Alveolar–Mixed Venous Tension Gradient

At the beginning of the alveolar uptake curve, the difference between the tension (partial pressure) of the anesthetic agent in alveolar gas and that in mixed venous blood is large. This gradient enhances the uptake of anesthetic by pulmonary blood and tends to slow the increase in alveolar concentration. As tissues and blood take up more anesthetic, this gradient decreases, and the effect of alveolar–mixed venous tension gradient on uptake is less obvious.

Second Gas Effect

In previous sections it has been assumed that the volatile anesthetic is delivered to the airway in oxygen only. If a high concentration of nitrous oxide is also added to the inspired mixture, the uptake of a large amount of this agent into blood will decrease the volume of the mixture in the alveoli, increase the alveolar concentration of the volatile agent, and "draw in" more anesthetic mixture from the upper airway. This phenomenon, called the second gas effect, is an additional factor that contributes to increasing the rate of alveolar uptake of a volatile agent whenever nitrous oxide is used.

Practical Implications

Of the factors mentioned, inspired concentration, alveolar ventilation, solubility in blood, and the second gas effect can be manipulated to promote alveolar uptake and increase the speed of induction. The inspired concentration can be set high initially; ventilation can be enhanced with assistance; and nitrous oxide can be added to the anesthetic mixture. Choosing a less soluble agent is attractive, but the choice is often limited by other considerations (e.g., unwanted side-effects).

Distribution and Tissue Uptake

Once an inhalation anesthetic is taken up by pulmonary blood, it is distributed to tissues of the body according to regional blood flow (see "Tissue Blood Flow and Tissue Mass" in Chap. 2). Tissues with the richest blood supply (brain, heart, liver, kidneys) take up the anesthetic rapidly. This rapid uptake of anesthetic by the brain means that its anesthetic partial pressure will very quickly come into equilibrium with that in the alveoli. This accounts for the popularity of the respiratory tract as a route for administration of anesthetic drugs.

Elimination

Excretion

Most of the inhalation agents are exhaled unchanged by the lungs. The fall in alveolar concentration follows an exponential decay curve (Fig. 3–4). The factors that influence this decay in alveolar concentration are exactly those that influence uptake, but the direction of the changes is reversed. Hyperventilation, a small FRC, a low solubility, a low cardiac output, or a large mixed venous–alveolar tension gradient increases the rate of decay. (Notice that "venous-alveolar" gradient instead of "alveolar-venous" gradient is used during excretion.) Hypoventilation, a large FRC, a high solubility, a large cardiac output, or a small mixed venous–alveolar tension gradient decreases the rate of this decay. Since

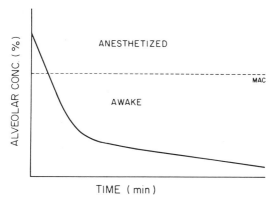

FIGURE 3–4. The fall in alveolar concentration of an inhalation anesthetic during emergence.

the inspired concentration of the agent is near zero during excretion, this factor has no influence on the rate of alveolar decay.

Metabolism

Until the mid-1960s it was believed that all inhalation anesthetics were exhaled unchanged. Since then, it has been observed that a significant portion of these inhaled agents is metabolized by mixed-function oxidases (the cytochrome P450 system) in the liver. The degree of biotransformation varies according to the agent, and most of the water-soluble organic and inorganic metabolites are excreted by the kidneys. The significance of these findings for individual agents is discussed in the following section.

SPECIFIC AGENTS

Nitrous Oxide

Nitrous oxide is a colorless, odorless, and nonflammable gas approximately 1½ times as heavy as air. It exists as a gas at room temperature and atmospheric pressure, but it can be compressed into a liquid unless its temperature is above 36.5° C. Medical-grade nitrous oxide is stored in cylinders as a liquid at room temperature under a pressure of 750 pounds per square inch (psi), or 50 atmospheres.

This agent is a weak anesthetic. Its MAC is 104%, a value that can be achieved only in the hyperbaric chamber. Normally no more than 70% nitrous oxide is administered in clinical practice, the other 30% being oxygen. After induction of anesthesia with an intravenous agent, it is given with a narcotic analgesic and a muscle relaxant to maintain anesthesia in the so-called balanced anesthesia technique. It is also used in combination with the more potent volatile agents. Since the MACs of nitrous oxide and other inhalation agents are additive (see "Minimum Alveolar Concentration," above), the use of nitrous oxide will reduce both the requirement of these agents and their side-effects. In contradistinction to its weak anesthetic property, nitrous oxide is a good analgesic. Premixed 50% nitrous oxide in oxygen (Entonox) is used for pain relief in obstetrics and in dental surgery.

Few side-effects are attributed to nitrous oxide. It does depress respiratory and myocardial function, but the degree of depression is small. Teratogenic effects have been observed in rats, and an increased incidence of spontaneous abortion has been reported in women who are chronically exposed to traces of nitrous oxide (e.g., operating room nurses and dental assistants). Administration of nitrous oxide for several days to patients during treatment of tetanus and poliomyelitis has also resulted in bone marrow depression and agranulocytosis.

Nitrous oxide is the only inorganic gas used in anesthesia today. It is not metabolized to any significant extent in the body.

Halothane

Halothane is a volatile, colorless, nonflammable liquid that is delivered by a calibrated vaporizer in clinical use. Its vapor has a pleasant odor, and its MAC is 0.77%. Despite its anesthetic potency, it is a poor analgesic. At anesthetic and subanesthetic doses, it reduces cerebral metabolism but increases cerebral blood flow and raises intracranial pressure.

Respiratory depression is a major side-effect of halothane and other volatile agents. Both the central chemoreceptor reflex (increase in ventilation in response to hypercapnia) and the peripheral chemoreceptor reflex (increase in ventilation in response to hypoxemia) are depressed. Patients anesthetized with halothane breathe with a distinct pattern that is fast but shallow. As a result, $PaCO_2$ is elevated, but severe hypercapnia is seldom a problem. Halothane can also cause bronchodilation; for this reason, it has been recommended as the agent of choice for patients with asthma or chronic bronchitis.

Nodal rhythm and a fall in arterial blood pressure are commonly seen during halothane anesthesia. Hypotension is particularly marked when halothane is given together with d-tubocurarine. The mechanism of its hypotensive effect is probably a combination of peripheral vasodilation, myocardial depression, depression of the vasomotor center, sympathetic ganglionic blockade, and inhibition of the baroreceptor reflex. (When baroreceptor reflex is depressed, vasoconstriction and tachycardia in response to a fall in blood pressure are inhibited.)

Another prominent cardiac side-effect of halothane is ventricular irritability. This problem is especially serious if the surgical field is infiltrated with epinephrine for hemostasis. It is recommended that the dose of epinephrine be limited to 10 ml of a 1:100,000 concentration in short procedures or to 30 ml of the same concentration in 1 hour during halothane anesthesia. Other factors that increase the incidence of ventricular arrhythmias during halothane anesthesia are surgical stimulation and hypercapnia. This increase in ventricular excitability can usually be controlled by an adequate depth of anesthesia and analgesia, by replacing part of the halothane with nitrous oxide, and by assisting the patient's ventilation. If ventricular arrhythmia remains troublesome despite the above remedies, halothane should be replaced with one of the other volatile agents.

Another important side-effect of halothane is its action on the gravid uterus. At anesthetic concentrations it can cause uterine relaxation, decrease the response of uterine muscle to oxytocin, and increase the incidence and severity of postpartum hemorrhage. Therefore only subanesthetic concentrations (no more than 0.5%) should be used for obstetric patients, except when relaxation of the uterus is desirable (e.g., for external version or delivery of retained placenta).

Halothane is still a popular inhalation agent in use today. Approximately 20% of the dose taken up by the body is metabolized in the liver in humans; the rest is exhaled unchanged. The water-soluble metabolites (bromide, chloride, and trifluoroacetic acid) are excreted in urine. For nearly 40 years it has been a safe and dependable agent, except for a rare and somewhat ill-defined sequela known as "halothane hepatitis," a syndrome characterized by postoperative fever, eosinophilia, and hepatic dysfunction with or without jaundice. The incidence is said to be higher with repeated exposures, particularly when they are close in time. It is recommended that patients not be exposed to halothane again for at least *3 months* after a halothane anesthetic.

Enflurane

Enflurane is another volatile, nonflammable liquid with a pleasant odor, but it is slightly more irritating to the upper airway than halothane. Its MAC is 1.7%. Enflurane has gained popularity in clinical practice because of the concern over halothane hepatitis following repeated exposure. Pharmacologically the two agents are very similar, except for the following differences:

1. Enflurane is less soluble in blood than halothane, so induction of and emergence from anesthesia are slightly more rapid with enflurane.

2. Under enflurane anesthesia approximately 2% of patients exhibit EEG patterns of seizure activity with or without muscle twitches, particularly in the presence of hypocapnia. The significance of these findings is unclear, but enflurane is not contraindicated for epilepsy patients.

3. Enflurane produces a useful degree of muscle relaxation and reduces the required dose of nondepolarizing muscle relaxants.

4. Ventricular arrhythmias are much less common with enflurane than with halothane, and interaction with epinephrine is highly variable.

5. Enflurane has a somewhat more potent circulatory and a considerably more potent respiratory depressant effect than halothane at equivalent anesthetic concentrations.

6. Only 2–4% of enflurane taken up by the human body is metabolized. Metabolism results in a low serum concentration of inorganic fluoride, which is potentially nephrotoxic. This is of little

clinical significance except in patients whose renal function is already impaired.

Isoflurane

Isoflurane, the latest volatile agent introduced into anesthetic practice, has an MAC of 1.15%. Its physical and pharmacologic properties are similar to those of halothane and enflurane, but it is distinguishable from the other two by the following qualities:

1. Of the three agents, isoflurane is the least soluble in blood, and alveolar uptake and washout are the most rapid.

2. The respiratory depressant action of isoflurane is somewhere between that of halothane and that of enflurane.

3. Isoflurane has the least potent myocardial depressant action. The drop in blood pressure seen in patients anesthetized with this agent is largely accounted for by a similar decrease in peripheral vascular resistance with little change in cardiac output. This property has made it nearly a perfect agent for inducing "controlled hypotension." It does not increase ventricular irritability and is compatible with infiltration of the surgical site with epinephrine. Isoflurane would have been the agent of choice for patients who have coronary artery disease, except for the observation that it can shunt coronary blood flow away from collateral-dependent ischemic regions (coronary steal). However there is no clear evidence that it does precipitate myocardial ischemia in these patients.

4. Among the volatile agents isoflurane causes the least increase in cerebral blood flow, and its vasodilating action on cerebral blood vessels is effectively blocked by simultaneous hyperventilation. This makes isoflurane the preferred agent in neurosurgical anesthesia.

5. Isoflurane produces better muscle relaxation than enflurane.

6. Isoflurane is more resistant to metabolic breakdown than halothane or enflurane. Less than 1% of the dose taken up by the body is metabolized.

7. No clear evidence of hepatotoxicity or nephrotoxicity attributable to isoflurane has been reported to date.

Methoxyflurane

Among the modern inhalation agents, methoxyflurane is the least volatile and the most soluble in blood. It is also, by far, the most potent, its MAC being 0.16%. Approximately 50% of the dose taken up by the body is metabolized. A small but significant number of patients (three in 10,000) develop renal failure characterized by a large urine volume following methoxyflurane anesthesia. Renal toxicity is dose related and is enhanced by other drugs that induce proliferation of liver enzymes (e.g., alcohol and tranquilizers) and those that can cause renal impairment (e.g., tetracycline). Its nephrotoxic action is attributed to a high serum level of inorganic fluoride, a product of biotransformation of methoxyflurane. For this reason, it has been largely supplanted by other agents. However it is also a potent analgesic; subanesthetic concentrations of this agent are still employed in some obstetric units to provide analgesia during labor.

Agents Under Investigation

Sevoflurane.   Sevoflurane is a nonflammable, insoluble agent (blood-gas partition coefficient, 0.69). It is being reinvestigated because of continued interest in rapid-acting agents. Its projected MAC in man is 2.6%, and its pharmacologic properties are similar to those of the other volatile agents. Onset of anesthesia is associated with depression of ventilation and blood pressure. Although it has promising characteristics, the fact that it undergoes extensive biotransformation in the body and can react with soda lime to produce potentially toxic products has prevented its release for clinical use so far.

I-653.   This highly volatile, insoluble agent is structurally similar to isoflurane. Having a blood-gas partition coefficient (0.42) similar to that of nitrous oxide, it is compatible with rapid induction and recovery and is ideal for outpatient surgery. It is also resistant to metabolic transformation, but it is not a potent agent. Its projected MAC in man is 5.6%.

Narcotic Analgesics

Crude opium has been used medicinally since biblical times, mainly for its antidiarrheal effect. Morphine, a pure opioid alkaloid, was not isolated until 1803 and has since been exploited for its antidiarrheal, antitussic, and analgesic properties. The opioids are narcotic analgesics; their principal application in the practice of anesthesia today is to relieve pain, either during the operation or in the postoperative period. Since the 1970s, large doses of opioids (mainly morphine and the fentanyls) have also been used to induce and maintain anesthesia in patients undergoing cardiac operations and in those who are critically ill.

MORPHINE

Mechanism of Action

The discovery of opioid receptors in the early 1970s expanded our knowledge of pain and its treatment. These receptors are widely scattered throughout the entire central nervous system, but they are more concentrated in the limbic system, the thalamus and hypothalamus, the striatum, the reticular activating system in the mid-brain, and the substantia gelatinosa of the spinal cord. Morphine interacts with these receptors to produce all its observed central effects. There are also endogenous polypeptides that can interact with these receptors to produce effects not unlike those of morphine; these are the *enkephalins* and the *endorphins*. It is postulated that the analgesic action of morphine and other opioids is the consequence of interaction between the compounds and the opioid receptors, which leads to inhibition of neurotransmitter release by afferent pain fibers.

There are at least four species of opioid receptors, each of which is responsible for the expression of specific characteristics: the μ-receptors for supraspinal analgesia, respiratory depression, euphoria, and physical dependence; the κ-receptors for spinal analgesia, miosis, and sedation; the σ-receptors for dysphoria, hallucination, and cardiac stimulation; and the δ-receptors for changes in affective behavior. Morphine, an *agonist*, acts primarily on the μ-receptors and to a lesser extent, on the κ-receptors. Some compounds exert only limited morphine-like actions; they are *partial agonists*. Other compounds compete with morphine for these receptors but exert no morphine-like actions; they are *competitive antagonists*. Still others exert antagonist-like actions at the μ-receptors and agonist-like actions at the κ- and σ-receptors; they are *agonist-antagonists*.

Systemic Effects

Central Nervous System.   The effects of morphine on the central nervous system are both depressive and stimulatory. Depression leads to analgesia, sedation, mood changes, and alveolar hypoventilation. Stimulation leads to pupillary constriction, nausea and vomiting, hyperactive spinal reflexes, and convulsions.

Many central nervous system depressants can produce a state of analgesia, but only together with gross impairment of intellectual function or unconsciousness. Morphine and other opioids, on the other hand, are selective analgesics because they can produce profound analgesia with little sedation and no effects on other sensory modalities. After an analgesic dose of morphine, most patients who are experiencing pain will feel relaxed, tranquil, and drowsy, provided nausea or vomiting is not a problem. However morphine alone is a poor anesthetic and a poor amnestic agent; many patients who had ultrahigh doses of morphine for anesthesia could recall intraoperative events vividly.

Alveolar hypoventilation is a result of the direct action of morphine on respiratory centers at the brain stem. The degree of respiratory depression is dose related. Death from an overdose is invariably due to respiratory failure. Even after a therapeutic dose, responsiveness of the respiratory centers to a rise in $PaCO_2$ is obtunded. While tidal volume remains relatively unchanged, respiratory rate is diminished and minute volume is reduced. Suppression of the cough reflex and decreased frequency of sighing are also part of this depression. Maximal respiratory effects occur between 5 and 10 minutes after an intravenous dose and between 30 and 60 minutes after an intramuscular dose. Therefore morphine is contraindicated in patients with respiratory insufficiency, unless artificial ventilation is instituted.

Pupillary constriction is an unmistakable side-effect of morphine, and pinpoint pupils are the hallmark of an overdose. Miosis is due to stimulation of the parasympathetic component of the third cranial (oculomotor) nerve nucleus. Morphine also directly stimulates the chemoreceptor trigger zone at the medulla, causing nausea and vomiting. This unpleasant side-effect is often delayed and is potentiated by ambulation. Truncal rigidity, a result of hyperactive spinal reflexes, is seen occasionally following intravenous administration of morphine and frequently following administration of fentanyl, but convulsion occurs with extremely high doses of morphine only.

Cardiovascular System. Morphine does not depress myocardial contractility, and therapeutic doses have little effect on hemodynamic function in young healthy adults when they are lying supine. However morphine is a potent dilator of resistance and capacitance vessels (arterioles and veins), and orthostatic hypotension is a common side-effect in ambulatory patients. Its peripheral action is largely the result of histamine release.

Respiratory System. Besides its effects on the control of breathing (see "Central Nervous System," above), morphine can induce bronchial constriction, in part by histamine release. Although this is of no consequence in healthy persons, morphine is contraindicated in patients with asthma or bronchitis who are having an acute attack of bronchospasm. It should also be used cautiously in those whose respiratory disease is in remission.

Gastrointestinal Tract. Morphine stimulates the smooth muscle of the gastrointestinal tract, but propulsive peristalsis is diminished and segmental tonic contraction is increased. The consequence is an increase in bowel transit time and constipation. Owing to spasm of Oddi's sphincter, pressure in the biliary tree can rise substantially after the administration of morphine. Many patients with gallbladder disease develop biliary colic after a therapeutic dose of morphine; this phenomenon can occur even years after cholecystectomy. The sudden onset of pain in these patients may be confused with acute myocardial ischemia. The spasm can be reversed by administration of naloxone or nitroglycerin, but only partially by administration of atropine.

Genitourinary Tract. Therapeutic doses of morphine increase contractions of the lower third of the ureter. This is of little clinical significance, though spasm of the bladder sphincter can lead to urinary retention.

Other Effects. Morphine has no direct effects on cerebral circulation, but hypercapnia following a therapeutic dose of morphine can increase cerebral blood flow and cause a rise in intracranial pressure in patients with intracranial space-occupying lesions. Furthermore the sedative and pupillary effects of morphine can interfere with assessment of neurologic functions in these patients. Therefore morphine and morphinelike opioids are not popular for neurosurgery.

It is said that therapeutic doses of morphine stimulate the release of antidiuretic hormone (ADH) and inhibit the stress-induced release of adrenocorticotropic hormone (ACTH). These observations are of little clinical significance.

Tolerance and Addiction. Tolerance to a drug is characterized by the need for increasing doses to obtain the same therapeutic effect after repeated exposure. Tolerance to morphine is obvious only with its depressant effects (e.g., analgesia and respiratory depression) and not with its excitatory effects (e.g., pupillary constriction and constipation). Tolerance to morphine is a reversible phenomenon, and sensitivity to a therapeutic dose will return to normal after 1–2 weeks' abstinence. Despite differences in molecular structure, cross-tolerance occurs between morphine and other opioid agonists. The mechanisms of tolerance and cross-tolerance are unclear.

Addiction is a state of psychological and physical dependence that manifests itself in the withdrawal syndrome. Mild physical dependence can occur as early as 24 hours after the first dose of morphine if it is given regularly (e.g., for pain in the immediate postoperative period). Signs of withdrawal usually appear approximately 8 hours after the last dose. They are mild at first, and the patient appears anxious and restless. The syndrome progresses over the next several hours, reaches a peak in 48–72 hours, and runs its course in 5–10 days. It is characterized by lacrimation, rhinorrhea, diaphoresis, vomiting and diarrhea, incessant yawning, gooseflesh, dilated pupils, hypertension, tachycardia, abdominal cramps, and muscle aches. Cross-dependence between morphine and other opioid agonists can occur. The administration of an opioid antagonist to patients addicted to morphine or other agonists will precipitate this syndrome. The mechanism of addiction, like that of tolerance, is not known.

Drug Interaction.   Phenothiazines counteract the emetic effect of morphine but potentiate its analgesic, sedative, and respiratory depressant effects. Similarly the depressive effects on respiratory centers caused by opioid agonists and those caused by intravenous and inhalation anesthetics are additive.

Allergy and Idiosyncrasy.   Allergic reactions to morphine are rare. Wheals and itching at the site of injection are local reactions to histamine release and should not be considered signs of true allergy. Many patients regard nausea and vomiting following morphine injection as an allergic manifestation. Careful questioning will reveal details of the event so that these reactions can be confirmed to be mere side-effects.

Uptake, Distribution, and Fate

In anesthesia practice morphine is given subcutaneously, intramuscularly, or intravenously. Approximately 60% of a subcutaneous dose is absorbed within 30 minutes after injection. Absorption from intramuscular sites is even faster. After absorption, approximately a third of the drug appearing in plasma is protein bound. Only a small quantity of the free fraction crosses the blood-brain barrier to act on opioid receptors; the rest is taken up by skeletal muscle, the lungs, and other visceral organs.

The major pathways for elimination of morphine from the body are conjugation in the liver with glucuronic acid and excretion of the water-soluble metabolite by the kidneys. Nearly 90% of an injected dose is recovered in urine within 24 hours. The other 10% is excreted in bile and appears in feces.

Application in Anesthesia Practice

Morphine is the most popular opioid used in all aspects of anesthesia care of the surgical patient. In combination with a parasympatholytic agent (e.g., atropine or hyoscine) or a phenothiazine (e.g., chlorpromazine or prochlorperazine), it is useful as a preanesthetic sedative. In the operating room, it is given intravenously as an analgesic adjuvant to general anesthesia. By far the most popular use of morphine in surgical patients is to relieve pain. In this respect morphine is prescribed on the basis that it is given only when necessary. For pain of moderate intensity, a dose of 10–15 mg given subcutaneously or intramuscularly every 4 hours is usually adequate in adults. If pain is severe, the intravenous route is recommended; increments of 1–2 mg may be given as required. It must be stressed that the analgesic dose of opioids varies according to the intensity of pain; dose should be titrated against effect. (Oxymorphone and hydromorphone are semisynthetic derivatives of morphine. Their pharmacologic actions are similar to those of the parent compound, but they are 8–10 times more potent.)

OTHER OPIOIDS

Agonists

Papaveretum. Papaveretum is a mixture of purified opium alkaloids, of which 50% is morphine. Its actions and fate are similar to those of its major component. Satisfactory pain relief can be obtained with a dose of 10–20 mg given subcutaneously or intramuscularly every 4 hours or 2–4 mg given intravenously when necessary.

Meperidine. Meperidine is a synthetic agent whose molecular formula is quite different from that of morphine, but the actions and side-effects of the two agents are quite similar, except that

1. Meperidine has atropine-like effects that include dry mouth and blurred vision.
2. Fewer patients given meperidine are troubled with consti-

pation. Its spasmogenic effect on the biliary tract and Oddi's sphincter is also less.

3. Pupillary constriction following an equianalgesic dose of meperidine is not as marked as that after morphine.

4. It has been demonstrated to be the most effective agent in stopping postoperative shivering.

5. Unlike morphine, large doses of meperidine have a discernible depressant effect on myocardial function. An increase in heart rate following intravenous injection of meperidine is also common.

6. The duration of action of meperidine is shorter than that of morphine.

This opioid is transformed in the liver by hydrolysis, conjugation, and demethylation. The products of detoxification are excreted in urine. Very little meperidine is excreted unchanged, but excretion of the unchanged fraction can be increased by acidification of urine (see ion trapping under "Physical Characteristics of the Drug" in Chap. 2).

Meperidine is only one-tenth as potent as morphine. For analgesia a dose of 75–125 mg is given intramuscularly every 3–4 hours, or 10–15 mg intravenously when necessary. Since meperidine can cause local irritation, it is not given subcutaneously.

Fentanyl and Its Congeners. *Fentanyl* is a synthetic agent related to meperidine. It is more lipophilic than morphine and crosses the blood-brain barrier with ease, thus accounting for the rapid onset and short duration of action. It is broken down by the liver, and the metabolites are excreted in urine.

The degree and duration of respiratory depression following fentanyl are dose related, but the respiratory depressant effect may last longer than its analgesic action. Truncal rigidity following intravenous administration of large doses is a common observation, but signs of histamine release are rare. This opioid is free of circulatory depressant effects, though bradycardia can occur with very large doses.

Fentanyl is 100 times more potent than morphine, and its duration of analgesic action after a single intravenous dose of 1.5 μg/kg is approximately 30 minutes. Owing to this short duration of action, fentanyl is not useful by injection for treatment of pain that is persistent; it is more useful either as an analgesic supplement during surgery or as a total anesthetic (together with oxygen and a muscle relaxant) in cardiac surgery. In the former case, 1–3 μg/kg is given initially, and 25 μg subsequently every 30 minutes when required. In the latter case, 50–150 μg/kg is given slowly for induction and maintenance of anesthesia. Intraoperative awareness has not been reported with doses larger than 120 μg/kg, but hypertension in reaction to surgical stimuli can still occur. The pressor response can be attenuated by using a hypotensive agent (e.g., nitroglycerin), small doses of diazepam, or low concentrations of a volatile anesthetic. A common problem seen with induction doses of fentanyl is the development of truncal rigidity before loss of consciousness. This reaction can be abolished by giving a small dose of muscle relaxant and instituting manual ventilation of the lungs.

Precautions. Fentanyl and all its congeners are potent respiratory depressants. Transient apnea requiring assisted ventilation is not uncommon when analgesic doses are given to patients who are breathing spontaneously. When anesthetic doses are used, controlled ventilation should continue well into the postoperative period, until the patient has recovered from the respiratory depressant effect.

Sufentanil is seven to ten times as potent as fentanyl. It is more effective than the parent compound in blocking the pressor response to noxious stimuli and has a better margin of safety (therapeutic index). The pharmacologic properties of the two congeners are similar but sufentanil appears to have a more pronounced negative inotropic effect on the heart. It is also a more potent respiratory depressant, and instances of patients remaining apneic after regaining consciousness have been observed.

Sufentanil is broken down in the liver and small intestine by oxidative dealkylation into inactive metabolites that are excreted in urine and feces. Since elimination is rapid and accumulation in tissue stores is limited, recovery is faster with sufentanil than with fentanyl. It is also employed in surgery both as an analgesic supplement and as a complete anesthetic. When it is used to supplement anesthesia, 0.2–0.7 μg/kg should be given at the beginning of surgery to be followed by increments of 5–10 μg when required. In cardiac surgery, 8–30 μg/kg is given slowly during induction together with oxygen and a muscle relaxant.

Alfentanil is the newest congener that is one-fifth to one-third as potent as fentanyl. It is extensively metabolized in the liver and small intestine and is eliminated from the body even faster than sufentanil. Hence times to awakening, orientation, and ambulation following a therapeutic dose of alfentanil are significantly shorter than those following an equipotent dose of fentanyl or sufentanil. It is given in incremental doses or in continous infusion to supplement oxygen-nitrous oxide anesthesia. When the operation is not expected to exceed 30 minutes, 5–20 μg/kg should be given initially, followed by increments of 2.5 μg/kg as required. The total dose should be limited to 5–40 μg/kg. When surgery is expected to last between 30 and 60 minutes, 20–50 μg/kg should be given at the beginning, followed by increments of 5–15 μg/kg when indicated. The total dose should not exceed 75 μg/kg. When a continuous infusion is contemplated for operations longer than 45 minutes, a loading dose of 50–75 μg/kg should be given at the beginning, to be followed by an infusion of 0.5–1.5 µg/kg/min. In the last two instances, endotracheal intubation with controlled ventilation is recommended.

Codeine.   Codeine is another naturally occuring opium alkaloid. When given parenterally its analgesic potency is only one-sixth to one-tenth that of morphine. However it is widely used as an oral analgesic (in combination with acetylsalicylate or acetaminophen) because (when compared to other opioids) only a relatively small fraction of codeine in portal venous blood is cleared by the liver immediately following enteric absorption (first-pass hepatic clearance). In fact, part of the codeine in portal venous blood is converted to morphine in the liver. Eventually elimination of codeine is by conjugation in the liver and by excretion of water-soluble metabolites in urine.

An analgesic dose of codeine has little effect on mental state, pupil size, and respiration. This lack of side-effects is a distinct advantage in neurosurgical and ambulatory patients. Otherwise use of codeine parenterally for analgesia is not popular. Usually a dose of 30–60 mg is given subcutaneously or intramuscularly every 3–4 hours for the treatment of pain following surgery. This dose can also be given orally for minor pain. (Oxycodone and hydrocodone are semisynthetic derivatives of codeine. While oxycodone is formulated with acetylsalicylate or acetaminophen and used as an oral analgesic, hydrocodone is employed only in antitussive medications.)

Alphaprodine.   Alphaprodine is another synthetic agent that resembles meperidine in pharmacologic actions but has an even shorter duration of action (1–2 hours following subcutaneous injection). Usually a dose of 5–10 mg is given intravenously when necessary to supplement general anesthesia.

Agonist-Antagonists

Pentazocine.   Pentazocine was synthesized in the 1960s during a search for a potent analgesic without addictive properties. It is an agonist-antagonist with potent agonist but mild antagonist actions. It differs from morphine in the following ways:

1. The degree of respiratory depression produced by an analgesic dose of pentazocine is similar to that produced by an equianalgesic dose of morphine, but increasing the dose of pentazocine does not produce further respiratory depression. This limited degree of respiratory depression is seen with three other agonist-antagonists: *nalbuphine, butorphanol, and buprenorphine*.

2. In general the stimulatory actions of pentazocine on smooth muscle of the gastrointestinal tract are much milder than those of morphine.

3. Unlike morphine, pentazocine given intravenously can produce a rise in systemic and pulmonary arterial pressures as well as elevation of left ventricular end-diastolic pressure. Its circulatory depressant effect is particularly obvious in patients with heart disease.

4. Being an agent with mild antagonist actions, pentazocine can precipitate withdrawal syndrome in patients addicted to morphine or other opioids.

5. Dysphoria is a frequent side-effect of pentazocine.

Owing to its low potential for abuse, the main application of pentazocine is in the treatment of chronic pain. It has also been used for premedication and as an analgesic supplement in general anesthesia. A dose of 30–60 mg is given subcutaneously or intramuscularly every 3–4 hours. This agent is also effective in the treatment of minor surgical pain when given orally; the usual adult dose is 50 mg every 4 hours after meals.

Antagonists

Naloxone. The original "antagonists" used in anesthesia practice, *nalorphine* and *levallorphan*, are in fact agonist-antagonists. Naloxone, on the other hand, is a pure opioid antagonist. Although it is devoid of morphine-like agonist activities, it promptly reverses the morphine-like actions of all opioids and precipitates a full-blown withdrawal syndrome in addicts. Following administration of naloxone to patients who have received a therapeutic dose of morphine, respiratory rate increases, drowsiness disappears, pupils dilate, Oddi's sphincter relaxes, and blood pressure, if depressed, returns to normal. Likewise, naloxone reverses the agonist actions of pentazocine, butorphanol, and nalbuphine. In addition to these specific antagonist actions, naloxone also has a mild, nonspecific action on the central nervous system and partially reverses the depressant effects of pentobarbital and diazepam. This agent is poorly absorbed via the gastrointestinal tract and must be given by injection. It is metabolized in the liver, chiefly by conjugation with glucuronic acid.

The major indication for naloxone is in the treatment of excessive respiratory depression induced by opioids. The dose is 100 µg to be given intravenously and repeated when necessary (10 µg/kg in neonates and infants). Its effect is obvious within 1–2 minutes following injection. With careful titration, it is possible to reverse excessive respiratory depression without depriving the patient of adequate analgesia. If the dose of naloxone is excessive, an "overshoot" phenomenon characterized by hyperpnea, agitation, and hypertension is seen. Therefore careful titration is mandatory. Since the duration of action of most opioids is longer than that of a single intravenous dose of naloxone, patients should be observed until the effect of the agonist has worn off.

Naltrexone.   This is a newer antagonist that is active following oral administration. It has a half-life of 10 hours, and the antagonist actions of a single oral dose can last up to 48 hours. It is currently under clinical trial; its long duration of action may prove to be an advantage.

Muscle Relaxants

All resting muscles have tone. There is a tendency for them to resist being stretched because small groups of muscle fibers are contracting at random; in fact they contract when stretched. If conduction of impulses in a motor nerve is interrupted, the muscle it innervates becomes flaccid. In the practice of anesthesia, muscle relaxation refers to the suppression of this resting muscle tone and stretch reflex. Usually only a mild degree of relaxation is required for operations on the body wall and extremities, but profound relaxation is required for operations within body cavities.

In the era of ether anesthesia, profound relaxation suitable for upper abdominal operations was obtained by increasing the depth of anesthesia to Plane 2 or 3 of Stage III (see "Stages of Ether Anesthesia" in Chap. 1). In current practice, use of muscle relaxant has allowed the anesthesiologist to obtain the desired degree of muscle relaxation without resorting to dangerous depression of the central nervous system. Since the introduction of curare nearly 50 years ago, many compounds of diverse origin have been found to possess muscle-relaxant properties. These compounds block the transmission of neural impulses between motor nerve endings and muscle fibers. In order to understand the mechanism of their action, it is necessary to review the sequence of events during normal neuromuscular transmission.

PHYSIOLOGY OF NEUROMUSCULAR TRANSMISSION

Anatomy of the neuromuscular junction and the physiology of neuromuscular transmission are summarized in Figure 5–1. The junction between the motor nerve ending and the motor end-plate—a thickened area of muscle membrane thrown into folds—is a specialized functional unit. Before a motor nerve approaches the end-plate region of the muscle fiber, it sheds its myelin sheath and divides into a number of terminal buttons. Each of these

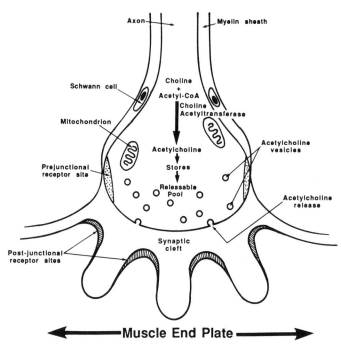

FIGURE 5–1. The neuromuscular junction with presynaptic and postsynaptic acetylcholine receptors.

buttons fits into a depression in the motor end-plate, but a discrete gap (the synaptic cleft) remains between nerve and muscle.

The chemical messenger traversing this cleft is acetylcholine. It is the product of acetylation of choline, a process catalyzed by the enzyme choline acetyltransferase. This transmitter substance is stored in clear vesicles, each of which has a discrete number of molecules called a quantum of acetylcholine. Approximately 20% of these vesicles are easily mobilized for release; the rest act as depots from which the readily available store is replenished.

Upon arrival of an impulse at the motor nerve ending, a fixed number of quanta of acetylcholine are released into the neuromuscular cleft by exocytosis (reverse pinocytosis). This process is facilitated by the influx of calcium ions during depolarization of the motor nerve. Following release, acetylcholine diffuses rapidly across the synaptic cleft to combine with stereospecific receptor molecules situated on the crest of the postsynaptic membranous folds. As a result of this transmitter-receptor interaction, sodium channels in the underlying membrane are opened and movement of sodium ions intracellularly generates a depolarizing potential called the "end-plate potential." The height of this end-plate potential is directly proportional to the quanta of acetylcholine released and the number of postjunctional receptors combined with acetylcholine molecules. The propagation of this end-plate potential to the adjacent muscle membrane generates an action potential if a critical value known as the "threshold potential" is reached. This wave of action potential then travels up and down the entire length of the muscle fiber, and muscle contraction ensues. Subsequently the released acetylcholine is hydrolyzed by acetylcholinesterase, and the muscle fiber relaxes.

In addition to postjunctional acetylcholine receptors on the motor end-plate, there are prejunctional acetylcholine receptors on the nerve membrane. When released acetylcholine molecules combine with these prejunctional receptors, mobilization of acetylcholine from the depot to join the readily available pool is facilitated. This function ensures a steady supply of acetylcholine for release during sustained tetanic contractions.

MECHANISM OF NEUROMUSCULAR BLOCKADE

Although there is evidence that muscle relaxants act on many sites at the neuromuscular junction to block impulse transmission, the major site of action is the cholinergic-nicotinic receptors on the motor end-plate. These agents are divided into two subgroups according to whether their mode of action is nondepolarizing neuromuscular blockade or depolarizing neuromuscular blockade.

Nondepolarizing Neuromuscular Blockade

Nondepolarizing muscle relaxants are capable of combining reversibly with postjunctional cholinergic-nicotinic receptors without opening sodium channels. Their competition with acetylcholine for nicotinic receptors reduces the number of these receptors accessible to acetylcholine molecules released by the motor nerve. As the concentration of relaxant molecules increases, the population of functioning receptors declines. Consequently the amplitude of the end-plate potential in response to the quanta of acetylcholine released by each nerve impulse falls. (The amplitude of the end-plate potential is directly proportional to the quanta of acetylcholine released and the number of receptors accessible to acetylcholine.) When more than 70% of the receptors are blocked, the end-plate potential in response to a single nerve impulse will not reach the threshold required to generate an action potential. Consequently the muscle fiber remains inert. However the muscle fiber still can respond to repetitive nerve impulses arriving at the motor nerve ending in quick succession, even at this level of neuromuscular blockade. As the population of the blocked receptors grows, an increasing number of muscle fibers fail to respond to nerve impulses. When 90–95% of the receptors are blocked, neuromuscular transmission fails completely and the muscle becomes flaccid. The method of evaluating the degree of nondepolarizing neuromuscular blockade is discussed in Chapter 14 (see "Monitoring Neuromuscular Function" and "Peripheral Nerve Stimulation").

Nondepolarizing muscle relaxants also can interfere with muscle contraction by their action on prejunctional receptors. Even in subparalyzing doses, these agents can competitively block the access of acetylcholine molecules to prejunctional receptors, interfering with mobilization of acetylcholine from storage depots and replenishment of the readily available pool. As a result, a steady demand for continuous release of acetylcholine cannot be sustained and tetanic contractions fade.

These actions of nondepolarizing relaxants can be reversed with anticholinesterases, which inhibit the hydrolysis of acetylcholine by acetylcholinesterase. Following administration of an anticholinesterase, the concentration of acetylcholine molecules at the neuromuscular junction rises. Since a higher concentration of acetylcholine can compete more effectively against relaxant molecules at both postjunctional and prejunctional receptor sites, neuromuscular transmission will return toward normal and tetanic contraction can be sustained once again. In practice it is recommended that an anticholinesterase should be given only after some spontaneous return of neuromuscular function is obvious; otherwise reversal of neuromuscular blockade may not be satisfactory.

Depolarizing Neuromuscular Blockade

Depolarizing muscle relaxants are also acetylcholine analogues; but unlike nondepolarizing agents, they have agonist activities. Interaction between these molecules and postjunctional cholinergic-nicotinic receptors depolarizes both the motor end-plate and the muscle fiber. Consequently the muscle contracts, although the contraction is not sustained. But as long as the receptors are occupied by these molecules, depolarization of the motor end-plates persists, neuromuscular transmission is interrupted, and the muscle remains flaccid. This is the *Phase I* depolarizing *block*. The hallmark of a depolarizing neuromuscular blockade is random contraction of motor units, seen as muscle fasciculations, followed by paralysis. The electromechanical characteristics of the Phase I depolarizing block are discussed in Chapter 14 (see "Peripheral Nerve Stimulation"). During Phase I block, mobilization of depot acetylcholine remains normal and no fade occurs during tetanic contraction.

Recovery from Phase I block depends on washout of relaxant molecules from the junctional area and their elimination from the body. Compared with nondepolarizing muscle relaxants, depolarizing agents are eliminated from the body more rapidly, and their action at the neuromuscular junction is short lived.

If Phase I block is maintained with continuous infusion or repeated injection of a depolarizing agent, both postjunctional and prejunctional receptors may become insensitive to the normal action of acetylcholine, even after the relaxant molecules are removed from the junctional area. This is *Phase II block*, also known as *dual block* or *desensitization block*. Phase II block has all the electromechanical characteristics of the nondepolarizing block (see "Peripheral Nerve Stimulation" in Chap. 14). Like the nondepolarizing block, a fully developed Phase II block can be reversed with anticholinesterases. The mode of action by which Phase II block is produced is unclear. Sensitivity of the receptors to acetylcholine usually returns with time.

NONDEPOLARIZING MUSCLE RELAXANTS

A large number of nondepolarizing muscle relaxants with varying properties and duration of action are available, but *d*-tubocurarine is still a standard to which all others are compared.

LONG-ACTING AGENTS

d-Tubocurarine

After intravenous injection, the action of *d*-tubocurarine reaches a peak in 4 minutes and lasts approximately 30–45 minutes. Adequate muscle relaxation can be obtained with a loading dose of 0.3–0.4 mg/kg and maintained with increments of 0.1 mg/kg when necessary. (Nondepolarizing blocks are potentiated by succinylcholine given previously to facilitate tracheal intubation and by volatile agents given concurrently. The dose of all nondepolarizing muscle relaxants recommended is based on these assumptions.)

A significant amount of circulating *d*-tubocurarine is bound to plasma protein (more to globulin than to albumin). Approximately 40% of an injected dose is recoverable in urine within 24 hours, a small amount is taken up by tissues, and the rest is eliminated via biliary excretion.

The most obvious side-effect of *d*-tubocurarine is arterial hypotension. The degree of hypotension is particularly severe in the elderly, in patients who are hypovolemic, and in those under halothane anesthesia. The fall in blood pressure is related chiefly to histamine release from tissue depots and partly to sympathetic ganglionic blockade.

Owing to its hypotensive side-effect and histamine-releasing property, *d*-tubocurarine should be administered with care to elderly or hypovolemic patients and to those with asthma and bronchitis. Otherwise there are few contraindications to its use, provided that artificial ventilation of the lungs is instituted.

Pancuronium

Pancuronium, a nonmetabolic steroid, is five times as potent as *d*-tubocurarine and has a slightly longer duration of action. Maximal muscle relaxation is seen within 2 minutes following intravenous injection. The recommended loading dose is 0.06–0.08 mg/kg. Increments of 0.01–0.02 mg/kg can be given when necessary.

A considerable amount of pancuronium is bound to plasma protein. Compared with *d*-tubocurarine, this agent is more dependent on renal excretion for elimination. As much as 80% of an injected dose is recoverable from the urine of laboratory animals; the rest is metabolized and excreted by the liver. Hepatic metabolism produces active but less potent metabolites that are of little clinical importance.

Sinus tachycardia with or without an increase in blood pressure is a common side-effect following the injection of a bolus of pancuronium. This pressor response is partly the result of a parasympatholytic action on the cardiac vagus and partly of the inhibition of catecholamine reuptake by sympathetic nerves. Unlike *d*-tubocurarine, pancuronium has no significant effect on autonomic ganglia and causes little histamine release. It is by far the most popular long-acting nondepolarizing muscle relaxant in current practice.

Metocurine

Metocurine is twice as potent as *d*-tubocurarine but has a similar duration of action. Optimal muscle relaxation can be obtained with a loading dose of 0.15–0.2 mg/kg and maintained with increments of 0.03 mg/kg when necessary. It has no effect on the sympathetic ganglia and is devoid of histamine-releasing properties, but it can still cause arterial hypotension in a significant number of patients. It is largely dependent on renal excretion for elimination and should not be given to patients with impaired renal function.

INTERMEDIATE-ACTING AGENTS

Gallamine

Gallamine is one-fifth as potent as d-tubocurarine. After intravenous injection, action reaches a peak between 2 and 3 minutes, and duration of action approaches 30 minutes. The recommended loading dose and increment for maintenance are 1.5–2 mg/kg and 0.5 mg/kg, respectively. Histamine release is considerably less with gallamine that with d-tubocurarine. The most prominent side-effect is sinus tachycardia, a result of cardiac vagal blockade. This agent is totally dependent on renal excretion for elimination and is absolutely contraindicated for patients in renal failure.

Atracurium

Atracurium is as potent as d-tubocurarine. A dose of 0.3–0.4 mg/kg should be given initially, to be followed by increments of 0.08–0.1 mg/kg when necessary. Peak action is reached within 2–5 minutes after a bolus, and total paralysis lasts 20–35 minutes. Because of its relatively short duration of action and lack of cumulative effect, atracurium is given as a continuous infusion as well (at a rate of 5–8 μg/kg/min). Histamine release causing hypotension has been reported occasionally, but this usually occurs after a very large bolus is administered.

At normal body temperature and pH, approximately 50% of a dose is broken down in plasma by nonspecific esterases and a nonenzymatic chemical process known as Hoffman elimination; less than 25% is dependent on renal excretion for elimination. One of the products of degradation is laudanosine, a neurotoxin with convulsant properties; however the plasma level of laudanosine is clinically insignificant, even after major operations lasting several hours.

Vecuronium

Like pancuronium, vecuronium is five times as potent as d-tubocurarine but it has a duration of action of only 25–40 minutes. The initial dose is 0.08–0.1 mg/kg, to be followed by increments of 0.01–0.015 mg/kg as required. Vecuronium does not release histamine, nor does it cause hypotension. Up to 35% of a given dose is recoverable from urine in man, and more than 50% is secreted in bile. Its duration of action may be prolonged in patients who have liver cirrhosis or obstructive jaundice.

OTHER AGENTS

Alcuronium is a semisynthetic agent available only in Europe. It is twice as potent as *d*-tubocurarine and has a slightly shorter duration of action. The recommended loading dose is 0.2 mg/kg. It is said to be free of most of the unwanted side-effects of *d*-tubocurarine, but it is excreted only in urine and should be avoided in patients with impaired renal function.

A concerted effort is being made to find nondepolarizing agents that are fast acting, have a shorter duration of action and no cardiovascular side-effects, and are less dependent on renal excretion for elimination. Several compounds are undergoing clinical trials at present. *Pipecuronium*, another nonmetabolic steroid, is six times as potent as *d*-tubocurarine. Although its molecular structure is related to that of pancuronium, it does not seem to cause tachycardia or hypertension. *Doxacurium* (BW A938U), an agent at least 10 times as potent as *d*-tubocurarine, also has no cardiovascular side-effects. Both agents have a duration of action similar to that of pancuronium and probably depend on renal excretion for elimination. *Mivacurium* (BW 1090U), on the other hand, is a short-acting agent. Being hydrolyzed by plasma cholinesterase, it can be given as a continuous infusion without cumulative effects.

REVERSING A NONDEPOLARIZING BLOCK

Neuromuscular function following administration of a nondepolarizing muscle relaxant recovers with time. The time course of recovery depends on redistribution of the agent in body water and its eventual elimination by metabolism and excretion. Since at physiologic pH, most of the muscle relaxant molecules are electrically charged, tissue uptake is slow and duration of action is governed chiefly by the pathways of elimination.

At the end of a surgical procedure, recovery of neuromuscular transmission following administration of a nondepolarizing muscle relaxant is usually not complete. Therefore it is necessary to terminate the action of the nondepolarizing muscle relaxant with an anticholinesterase—neostigmine, pyridostigmine, or edrophonium. Since anticholinesterases work at both the neuromuscular junction and muscarinic sites (chiefly organs innervated by the vagus), muscarinic side-effects of these agents should be blocked by administering a vagolytic agent (atropine or glycopyrrolate) at the same time.

Neostigmine and Atropine. A combination of neostigmine, 0.03–0.07 mg/kg (maximum dose 5 mg), and atropine, 0.02–0.03 mg/kg (maximum dose 2.4 mg), is the preparation most commonly used to reverse the action of a nondepolarizing muscle relaxant.

Both drugs are usually mixed in the same syringe and administered intravenously as a bolus. The action of atropine at muscarinic sites always precedes that of neostigmine, and gross disturbance of cardiac rate and rhythm following the administration of this mixture is uncommon. Reversal of neuromuscular blockade is usually seen within 5 minutes. In order to ensure that normal neuromuscular function has returned, the patient should be observed closely during this period (see "Monitoring Neuromuscular Function" in Chap. 14).

Pyridostigmine.   Pyridostigmine is an analogue of neostigmine. A dose of 10–20 mg is required to counteract the effect of a nondepolarizing muscle relaxant in most adults. Its onset of action is somewhat delayed and may take 15 minutes. It has a longer duration of action than neostigmine and produces milder muscarinic side-effects. It should be given with 0.6–1.2 mg of atropine.

Edrophonium.   In small doses, the effect of edrophonium in reversing the action of nondepolarizing muscle relaxants is transient. It can be sustained by increasing the dose to 0.5–1 mg/kg. Compared with neostigmine, it has a quicker onset of action and milder muscarinic side-effects.

Glycopyrrolate.   Glycopyrrolate is a potent antisialagogue with no action on the central nervous system and minimal effects on the cardiovascular system. Its action is longer lasting than atropine. In order to block the muscarinic effects of neostigmine effectively, it should be given in the ratio of one part by weight of glycopyrrolate to five parts of neostigmine.

FACTORS AFFECTING ACTION

The potency, duration of action, and ease of reversal of nondepolarizing muscle relaxants are known to be affected by many physiologic and pharmacologic factors. They include priming, age, hypothermia, acid-base homeostasis, electrolyte imbalance, renal failure, myasthenia gravis, the Eaton-Lambert syndrome, and drug interactions.

Priming

All nondepolarizing muscle relaxants require a latency of at least 2–3 minutes for peak action to develop. A subparalytic dose of these agents given before the loading dose can decrease the latency and increase the potency of their action. Herein lies the principle of priming. In practice, one tenth of the calculated loading dose is given 4 minutes before the full intubating dose. This technique does not work consistently in all patients, and sensitive patients may develop significant paralysis following the calculated priming dose.

Age

The development of the neuromuscular junction is incomplete in premature infants and neonates. Many clinicians have found that this group of patients is more sensitive to nondepolarizing muscle relaxants. On the other hand, geriatric patients have decreased muscle bulk and are more sensitive to the effects of nondepolarizing muscle relaxants than are young adults. Since the rate of elimination of nondepolarizing muscle relaxants (particularly pancuronium) is slower in elderly persons, the duration of action is generally longer as well.

Hypothermia

Hypothermic patients are said to be relatively resistant to the neuromuscular blocking action of nondepolarizing muscle relaxants; however the rate of elimination of these agents by the kidneys and liver is also slowed. Therefore duration of action is prolonged under hypothermic conditions.

Acid-Base Homeostasis

The mechanism of interaction between hydrogen ions and nondepolarizing muscle relaxants is unknown, but it is difficult to reverse the block of nondepolarizing muscle relaxants when the $PaCO_2$ is more than 50 mm Hg. That is, *respiratory acidosis* potentiates the actions of nondepolarizing relaxants. *Metabolic alkalosis* may potentiate the blockade of nondepolarizing agents also, but *metabolic acidosis* does not seem to pose the same problem.

Electrolyte Imbalance

Hypokalemia, particularly that of acute onset, potentiates neuromuscular blockade of nondepolarizing muscle relaxants and diminishes the ability of anticholinesterases to reverse a nondepolarizing neuromuscular block. This enhancement is related to changes in the resting potentials of excitable tissues (muscle and nerves) in the presence of hypokalemia.

Renal Failure

Gallamine, metocurine, and alcuronium are eliminated from the body by renal excretion. Renal failure prolongs the duration of their action, and the standard practice of re-establishing neuromuscular transmission with an anticholinesterase is inadequate. In the absence of renal function, recovery of neuromuscular function is totally dependent on the redistribution of these drugs in the body. Since tissue uptake of these highly charged molecules is slow, recovery from a normal dose can take days.

d-Tubocurarine and pancuronium, on the other hand, are eliminated via both the kidneys and the liver, but pancuronium is slightly more dependent on renal excretion than is d-tubocurarine. In the presence of renal failure, clearance of these two agents by the kidneys is diminished, but hepatic clearance continues unabated and may even be enhanced. Reversal of their effects with an anticholinesterase is usually successful, even in anephric patients. Since the renal excretion of all anticholinesterases is also diminished in renal failure, there is no danger that the effects of the relaxants will outlast those of the anticholinesterases, unless the patient has been given an overdose of d-tubocurarine or pancuronium.

Myasthenia Gravis

Patients with myasthenia gravis have a block at the neuromuscular junction similar to that seen following administration of curare. This block can be successfully reversed with anticholinesterases. Myasthenia gravis patients are extremely sensitive to the effects of nondepolarizing muscle relaxants and are resistant to the Phase I block of depolarizing muscle relaxants. Adequate muscle relaxation can usually be obtained in these patients without the use of a muscle relaxant, provided that their medication (usually pyridostigmine) is omitted on the day of the operation. The degree of relaxation can be increased even further by using inhalation agents with good muscle-relaxant properties (enflurane and isoflurane). If use of a nondepolarizing muscle relaxant is absolutely essential, only a small dose (one thirtieth to one tenth the normal dose) should be given. Use of a peripheral nerve stimulator to follow the time course of neuromuscular blockade in this instance is mandatory.

Eaton-Lambert Syndrome

In the Eaton-Lambert (myasthenic) syndrome, originally described in patients with oat cell carcinomas, release of acetylcholine at motor nerve endings is impaired. Affected patients are sensitive to the effects of both nondepolarizing and depolarizing muscle relaxants.

Drug Interaction

All volatile anesthetic agents can potentiate the action of nondepolarizing muscle relaxants, but enflurane and isoflurane are more potent than halothane in this respect. The mechanism of interaction is probably related to :

1. A decline in efferent impulses in motor nerves due to depression of the central nervous system.

2. An increase in delivery of relaxant molecules to skeletal muscles as a result of increased muscle blood flow.

3. Stabilization of muscle cell membrane by the anesthetic agent.

Succinylcholine, a depolarizing muscle relaxant usually given to facilitate tracheal intubation, can increase the block of a subsequent dose of nondepolarizing agents by 10–20%. Nondepolarizing muscle relaxants should be given only after the patient has shown signs of recovery from succinylcholine, and the dose should be modified accordingly.

Magnesium antagonizes the action of calcium at motor nerve endings and inhibits the calcium-mediated release of acetylcholine. Magnesium sulfate, an agent used in the treatment of seizures associated with toxemia of pregnancy, enhances the neuromuscular blockade of nondepolarizing muscle relaxants. Similarly calcium-channel blockers (e.g., verapamil) can potentiate the action of these agents.

Aminoglycosides exert an action similar to that of magnesium on prejunctional motor nerve endings and enhance the action of nondepolarizing muscle relaxants. Other antibiotics, by acting on the postjunctional membrane, have a similar effect. Antibiotic agents that have been reported to potentiate nondepolarizing blockade include clindamycin, colistin, gentamicin, kanamycin, lincomycin, neomycin, paromomycin, polymyxin A and B, streptomycin, tetracycline, and viomycin. In contrast to the drugs mentioned above, anticonvulsants (phenytoin and carbamazepine) can cause resistance to the action of nondepolarizing muscle relaxants.

DEPOLARIZING MUSCLE RELAXANTS

PHARMACOLOGY OF SUCCINYLCHOLINE

There are only two useful depolarizing muscle relaxants, and succinylcholine has been used largely to the exclusion of decamethonium. It is composed of two molecules of acetylcholine joined end-to-end and has a rapid onset of action that is obvious within one vein-to-muscle circulation time. It is most commonly used during induction of anesthesia to facilitate tracheal intubation. The normal intubating dose is 1 mg/kg.

The ester bond of succinylcholine is hydrolyzed rapidly by plasma cholinesterase (pseudocholinesterase). Therefore it is a short-acting agent. Following an intravenous injection, neuromuscular function returns in 3–5 minutes unless paralysis is sustained with an intravenous infusion of appropriate dilution (usually 500 mg in 500 ml of 5% dextrose solution). Phase II block is always a possible complication during prolonged infusion. In order to reduce the incidence of this complication, the total dose of succinylcholine should be limited to 500 mg, and the duration of infusion to 60 minutes.

SIDE-EFFECTS

Succinylcholine has several well-known side-effects. They include cardiac arrhythmias, salivation, muscle pain, and increases in intragastric pressure, intracranial pressure, intraocular pressure, and serum potassium concentration. Bradycardia and salivation are muscarinic side-effects and can be prevented or treated with a parasympatholytic agent. The rest are related to muscle fasciculation and are attenuated by precurarization.

Cardiac Arrhythmias

Although succinylcholine mimics the action of acetylcholine, *sinus bradycardia* following its administration is common only in children. Following an intubation dose, heart rate usually increases in adults, but bradycardia and transient asystole have been reported when administration is repeated within 10 minutes. This complication can be prevented by atropine, given either in the premedication or intravenously during induction of anesthesia. *Ventricular premature beats* have also been reported following administration of succinylcholine, but there are usually other precipitating factors (e.g., hypoxemia, hypercapnia, the administration of exogenous catecholamine, and inadequate depth of anesthesia).

Salivation

Owing to its muscarinic effect on the salivary glands, succinylcholine is a potent sialagogue. The secretion is usually watery and presents little problem. If it is deemed necessary, this side-effect can be blocked by the administration of atropine or glycopyrrolate.

Muscle Pain

The incidence of postoperative myalgia following a paralyzing dose of succinylcholine is as high as 90%. Pain is particularly severe in ambulatory and very muscular patients. Damage to muscle fibers during fasciculation has been suggested to be the cause of this unpleasant side-effect, and myoglobinemia and myoglobinuria have been observed in some patients.

Increased Intragastric Pressure

Succinylcholine can cause a rise in intragastric pressure. Its magnitude varies from patient to patient, and pressures great enough to cause regurgitation of stomach contents have been reported. Presumably the increase in pressure is related to fasciculation of the abdominal musculature.

Increased Intracranial Pressure

During light anesthesia succinylcholine may cause an increase in intracranial pressure in patients with decreased intracranial compliance. This is likely due to a combination of afferent cerebral stimulation via the muscle spindles and increased carbon dioxide production. Pretreatment with a small subparalytic dose of a nondepolarizing agent or concurrent administration of deep anesthesia will prevent a rise in intracranial pressure.

Increased Intraocular Pressure

Concurrent with the onset of fasciculation, intraocular pressure increases after administration of succinylcholine. This side-effect lasts for only 5 minutes and is due both to fasciculation of extraocular muscles and dilation of choroidal blood vessels. While this rise in intraocular pressure is of little significance in most patients, it can cause extrusion of intraocular contents (e.g., vitreous) in patients with an open wound of the eye.

Increased Serum Potassium Concentration

In most surgical patients there is a small rise in serum potassium concentration (approximately 0.5 mEq/L) following administration of succinylcholine. This increase is attributed to the flux of potassium ions escaping from skeletal muscle cells during fasciculation. However, a much larger rise in potassium concentration is seen in certain patients. Hyperkalemic cardiac arrest following the administration of succinylcholine has occurred in severely burned or injured patients (particularly within 1 week to 2 months after the initial trauma). Similarly, cardiac arrest has occurred in patients with neuromedical and neurosurgical disorders (usually in the first 6 months following onset of hemiplegia or paraplegia). A large increase in serum potassium concentration may be found also in uremic patients, patients with severe intra-abdominal sepsis, and patients suffering from peripheral vascular disease complicated by muscle wasting.

FACTORS AFFECTING ACTION

Many factors can affect the action, potency, and duration of action of succinylcholine. They include precurarization, self-taming, myotonia, myasthenia gravis, atypical plasma cholinesterase, and others.

Precurarization

Pretreatment of the patient with a subparalyzing dose of non-depolarizing muscle relaxant (e.g., 3 mg of *d*-tubocurarine, 20 mg of gallamine, or 1 mg of pancuronium) can attenuate but not abolish many of the unwanted side-effects of succinylcholine mentioned above. This technique is known as precurarization. Precurarization will certainly attenuate the severity of fasciculation and muscle pain as well as the rise in intragastric, intracranial, and intraocular pressures. However the effectiveness of precurarization in preventing hyperkalemia is questionable; at best it offers susceptible patients only partial protection against this potentially fatal complication. Precurarization also decreases the potency of succinylcholine and delays the onset of paralysis. In order to overcome these disadvantages of precurarization, the dose of succinylcholine should be increased to 1.5–2 mg/kg.

Self-Taming

Administration of 8–10 mg/kg of succinylcholine before the full intubating dose can attenuate muscle fasciculations seen with this agent. This technique is known as self-taming. It is not as effective as precurarization and does not diminish the incidence of succinylcholine-induced myalgia. Nor is there evidence to suggest that self-taming attenuates the other unwanted side-effects associated with succinylcholine.

Myotonia

Myotonia is an inability to relax a muscle after it contracts. It is seen in patients suffering from myotonia dystrophica (myotonia atrophica) and myotonia congenita. The former is the most common form of muscular dystrophy, but the latter is rare. Myotonic muscles are not relaxed by succinylcholine; instead they go into sustained contraction (contracture). Therefore succinylcholine is contraindicated in myotonic patients.

Myasthenia Gravis

Myasthenic patients are somewhat resistant to Phase I block and are more prone to develop Phase II block. In practice, however, little difficulty is associated with use of a single dose of succinylcholine for tracheal intubation in these patients.

Atypical Plasma Cholinesterase

Plasma cholinesterase is a glycoprotein synthesized in the liver. At least five genetic variants determined by genes at two different loci have been identified: the usual, the atypical, the fluoride-resistant, the silent, and the C_5 variant.

The *usual variant* (cholinesterase $^{usual}_{1st\,locus}$ or E_1^u) has a strong cholinesterase activity and is the most common. In persons homozygous for this variant ($E_1^u E_1^u$) hydrolysis of succinylcholine is rapid and its duration of action is limited to 5 minutes. As much as 80% of the enzyme activity of these normal persons is inhibited by dibucaine. This percentage of inhibition is called the *Dibucaine Number*. That is, plasma from homozygotes with the usual enzyme has a Dibucaine Number of 80.

The *atypical variant* (E_1^a) has weak cholinesterase activity. Succinylcholine is hydrolyzed very slowly in persons homozygous for this variant ($E_1^a E_1^a$), and a single intubating dose produces prolonged paralysis in these patients. Approximately one in 3000 patients is homozygous with the atypical enzyme. Paradoxically only 20% of the intrinsic activity of the atypical enzyme is inhibited by dibucaine; that is, plasma from homozygotes with the atypical enzyme has a Dibucaine Number of 20. A significant number of patients are heterozygotes ($E_1^u E_1^a$), having both usual and atypical enzymes. The Dibucaine Number of the plasma of such persons ranges from 30 to 70. The duration of action of succinylcholine in these heterozygotes is only moderately prolonged (increased to 10–20 minutes) and is of little clinical significance.

While the *fluoride-resistant variant* (E_1^f) has moderately reduced cholinesterase activity that is resistant to inhibition by fluoride ions, the *silent variant* (E_1^s) has extremely weak cholinesterase activity. Homozygotes with the fluoride-resistant enzyme ($E_1^f E_1^f$) are only moderately sensitive to succinylcholine, but those with the silent enzyme ($E_1^s E_1^s$) are extremely sensitive. Both variants are rare.

The C_5 *variant* is determined by a gene in the second locus (cholinesterase $_{2nd\,locus}$ or E_2). Being 30% more potent than the usual enzyme, it is of little clinical significance.

Other Factors

Many other factors have been observed to be associated with a reduction in plasma cholinesterase activity. They include advanced liver disease, hemodialysis, pregnancy, and the use of oral contraceptive agents, echothiophate (an anticholinesterase eye drop used in the treatment of glaucoma), neostigmine, and cytotoxic agents (e.g., cyclophosphamide). Although the reduction in enzyme activity can be marked, prolonged apnea is rare except in patients who are being treated with echothiophate, neostigmine, or cytotoxic agents.

Local Anesthetics

Local anesthetics are drugs that block impulse conduction in nerve fibers. Many substances have local anesthetic properties, but only those that produce a transient and completely reversible inhibition of impulse propagation are clinically useful.

Cocaine, the first local anesthetic discovered, is an alkaloid extracted from the leaves of *Erythroxylon coca*, a shrub that grows in the highlands of Peru and Bolivia. Although its numbing action was described earlier by von Anrep, it was used for the first time as a local anesthetic in 1884 by the Austrian ophthalmic surgeon Karl Koller, who used it topically by instilling it into the conjunctival sac.

Cocaine is toxic and addictive. In many ways its undesirable properties have been an impediment to the development of regional anesthesia (except for experiments with spinal anesthesia). A safer substitute came in the form of procaine in 1905. Lidocaine, the most popular agent in use today, was introduced in 1948.

ANATOMY OF THE PERIPHERAL NERVE

The cellular unit of the peripheral nerve is the neuron (Fig. 6–1*A*). It has a cell body and a long process called the "nerve fiber." (The nerve fiber can be either an axon or a dendrite.) All nerve fibers are ensheathed by Schwann cells (Schwann cell sheath or neurolemma). In unmyelinated nerves, approximately 5–20 of these nerve fibers are embedded in the cytoplasm of a single Schwann cell (Fig. 6–1*B*). In myelinated nerves, a substantial layer of myelin (transformed Schwann cell membrane) lies between the nerve fiber and the Schwann cell cytoplasm (Fig. 6–1*C*). This myelin sheath is not continuous along the entire length of the myelinated fiber; it is interrupted periodically at the nodes of Ranvier.

All large peripheral nerves have mixed sensory, motor, and autonomic functions. In a typical peripheral nerve, the fibers are

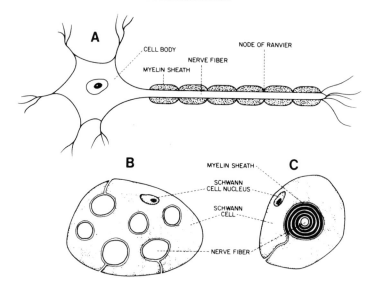

FIGURE 6–1.   Anatomy of the peripheral nerve. *A,* A typical neuron. *B,* Cross section of unmyelinated fibers. *C,* Cross section of a myelinated fiber.

bundled together to form fascicles, which in turn are bundled together to form the nerve trunk. The nerve trunk, the fascicles, and the nerve fibers are supported extensively by connective tissues known, respectively, as epineurium, perineurium, and endoneurium. Thus there are multiple barriers through which local anesthetics must travel to reach the neuronal membrane, the site of action.

PHYSIOLOGY OF IMPULSE CONDUCTION

The neuronal membrane is a bimolecular layer of phospholipids interspersed with globular protein molecules. It is normally freely permeable to positively charged potassium ions, relatively impermeable to positively charged sodium ions, and totally impermeable to negatively charged intracellular protein molecules. Within the membrane, there is also an energy-dependent membrane transport system that actively extrudes intracellular sodium in exchange for extracellular potassium. When the cell is at rest, the ratio of intracellular to extracellular potassium is 30:1 (150 mEq/L inside the cell and 5 mEq/L in the extracellular fluid). This excess of intracellular potassium is counterbalanced by a similar excess of extracellular sodium ions. However the electronegativity of intracellular protein molecules remains unchecked, and the nerve fiber has a resting membrane potential of -90 mV.

Following excitation (Fig. 6–2A), the sodium-potassium transport system of the neuronal membrane is paralyzed, permeability of the cell membrane to sodium ions increases, and movement of positively charged sodium ions into the cell through channels in the lipid membrane decreases the resting membrane potential (a process known as depolarization). When the transmembrane potential reaches -50 mV (the threshold potential), the sodium channels become fully open, so that the membrane is freely permeable to sodium ions. At this stage, sudden influx of positively charged sodium ions occurs, and the transmembrane potential rises rapidly to $+30$ mV. At the end of depolarization, sodium channels are closed again. Efflux of potassium ions restores the transmembrane potential to its resting value, and the cell is repolarized. Finally the sodium-potassium pump is reactivated and transmembrane gradients of potassium and sodium ions are restored. This wave of depolarization and repolarization is passed sequentially to adjacent points on the unmyelinated nerve fiber, and the impulse is propagated down its entire length. In myelinated fibers, the wave of excitation can skip from one node of Ranvier to the next (Fig. 6–2B), a phenomenon called "saltatory conduction." Therefore impulse propagation in myelinated fibers is much faster than that in unmyelinated fibers.

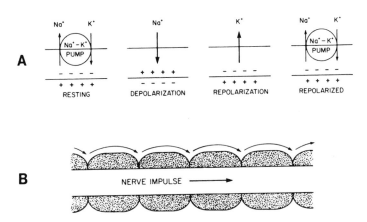

FIGURE 6–2.   Physiology of impulse conduction. *A*, The movement of sodium and potassium ions and local changes in electrical polarity during depolarization and repolarization. *B*, Saltatory conduction in a myelinated fiber.

MECHANISM OF LOCAL ANESTHETIC ACTION

Local anesthetics are lipophilic and weakly basic compounds available most commonly as water-soluble hydrochloride salts (XHCl). In aqueous solution they dissociate to form the respective base (X) and its acid (XH^+) according to the formulas:

$$XHCl \rightleftharpoons XH^+ + Cl^-$$
$$XH^+ \rightleftharpoons X + H^+$$

The existence of both species is necessary to explain the action of local anesthetics. The base, being nonionized, diffuses through tissue barriers readily, but it combines with a proton (H^+) to become the active acid on reaching the neuronal membrane. Since the pK_a of most local anesthetics lies between 7.5 and 9, the concentration of the ionized acid exceeds that of the nonionized base at tissue pH.

The mechanism of action of local anesthetics is not fully understood, but several hypotheses have been postulated to explain their action. They are the membrane receptor hypothesis, the membrane expansion hypothesis, and the surface charge hypothesis.

Membrane Receptor Hypothesis. As mentioned earlier, depolarization of the nerve fiber is the result of an influx of sodium ions into cells through channels in the membrane. The membrane receptor hypothesis proposes that local anesthetic molecules, by displacing calcium and binding receptors within these channels, block the influx of sodium ions and prevent depolarization and impulse propagation. Probably there is more than one receptor site within the sodium channels, but evidence suggests that all clinically useful agents act on receptors located on the inside surface of the neuronal membrane.

Membrane Expansion Hypothesis. The membrane expansion hypothesis postulates that presence of local anesthetic molecules in the lipid matrix of the neuronal membrane interferes with bonding of these lipid molecules and allows the membrane to expand. Expansion of the lipid matrix compresses sodium channels, blocks passage of sodium ions, and prevents depolarization and impulse propagation. This hypothesis is an extension of the lipid solubility hypothesis of general anesthesia and implies a single mode of action for both local and general anesthetics.

Surface Charge Hypothesis. The surface charge hypothesis proposes that negative charges on the external surface of the neuronal membrane are neutralized by the positively charged acid form of local anesthetic molecules without affecting the resting membrane potential (the potential difference between the interior and exterior of the nerve fiber). As a result, local current flow is disturbed, threshold of depolarization is increased, and propagation of nerve impulse is blocked.

SYSTEMIC EFFECTS OF LOCAL ANESTHETICS

The molecule of a typical local anesthetic has an aromatic (benzene) ring joined to a tertiary amine. If it is formed between an aromatic acid and an amino alcohol, the compound is an ester; if it is formed between an aromatic amine and an amino acid, the compound is an amide. Despite these differences both ester and amide compounds have similar pharmacologic actions and systemic side-effects.

Nerve Conduction

Nerve fibers have been classified into three groups according to their function and the degree of myelination: the A fibers of myelinated somatic nerves, the B fibers of myelinated preganglionic autonomic nerves, and the C fibers of nonmyelinated nerves. Furthermore the A fibers are subdivided into alpha, beta, gamma, and delta subgroups, according to their diameter: the largest are alpha fibers and the smallest, delta fibers. Transmission of pain and temperature is subserved by both the A delta fibers and the C fibers.

In general small and unmyelinated fibers are more sensitive to the action of local anesthetics, but there are exceptions. While the larger myelinated delta fibers and the small unmyelinated C fibers are equally sensitive, the myelinated B fibers are even more sensitive to the action of local anesthetic agents. Owing to the sensitivity of these autonomic fibers, sympathetic blockade following spinal or epidural anesthesia is more extensive than sensory blockade. This feature is responsible for the fall in blood pressure associated with these techniques.

When a local anesthetic is deposited around a nerve, it diffuses from the surface toward the core of the nerve trunk. Therefore conduction in mantle fibers (those on the surface) is blocked before that in core fibers. Since proximal parts of a limb are supplied by mantle fibers while distal parts are supplied by core fibers, it should not be surprising to find that anesthesia first develops proximally during a major nerve block (e.g., brachial plexus block).

Central Nervous System

Local anesthetics block impulse transmission in both peripheral nerves and the central nervous system. Fortunately central effects are seen only when plasma concentration has exceeded toxic levels (e.g., following an overdose or inadvertent intravenous injection). Since inhibitory pathways are depressed first, the initial clinical manifestation of central nervous system toxicity is a release phenomenon: excitation and convulsion. With even higher doses, all pathways are depressed, coma ensues, and death is usually due to respiratory arrest (see Chap. 17 for treatment of systemic toxicity).

Cardiovascular System

Most local anesthetics cause some degree of arteriolar dilation. In addition, all of them have direct effects on the myocardium. The myocardial effects of local anesthetics are best exemplified by those of lidocaine.

At therapeutic concentrations, lidocaine decreases the automaticity of Purkinje fibers exposed to a variety of arrhythmogenic stimuli. In this respect, lidocaine (1 mg/kg given as a bolus intravenously or 30 μg/kg/min given as an infusion) is useful in the treatment of ventricular arrhythmias. At toxic concentrations, however, it causes depression of myocardial excitability, conductivity, and contractility, all of which can lead to cardiovascular collapse and death.

Tachyphylaxis

Tachyphylaxis refers to the reduced potency of a local anesthetic agent when it is administered in repeated doses, as in continuous epidural anesthesia. This phenomenon is partly explained by an observed increase in hydrogen ion concentration locally after repeated administration of the acid salt. As tissue acidity increases, availability of the base form decreases (see "Mechanism of Local Anesthetic Action" above). Since only the uncharged base form can readily diffuse through tissue barriers, a decline in its concentration is seen clinically as reduced potency.

Hypersensitivity

Allergic reactions to local anesthetics, including dermatitis, bronchospasm, and anaphylaxis, have been reported from time to time. Most reports incriminate the ester-type agents. True hypersensitivity to local anesthetic agents may be extremely rare. Bacteriostatic additives may be responsible for some of the reported reactions.

ABSORPTION AND ELIMINATION

Systemic absorption of local anesthetic agents is determined by the site of injection, size of the dose, degree of protein binding, and pharmacologic characteristics of the agent. In addition, concomitant use of a vasoconstrictor (usually epinephrine 1:100,000) retards systemic absorption of local anesthetics; as a result, duration of action is prolonged, incidence of systemic toxicity reduced, and range of safe dose increased. After absorption, local anesthetics are distributed systemically according to regional blood flow. Ultimately they are eliminated from the body by metabolic degradation. Urinary excretion of unchanged drugs is relatively insignificant.

Ester-type compounds are hydrolyzed by esterase in the liver and by cholinesterase in the plasma. The degree and rate of hydrolysis by plasma cholinesterase vary according to the agent, being most marked for chloroprocaine, less for procaine, and least for tetracaine. It has been suggested that the rate of elimination of these agents may be prolonged in patients with atypical plasma cholinesterase. It is also suggested that procaine, by competing for plasma cholinesterase, can prolong the action of succinylcholine in normal persons.

Unlike ester-type compounds, amide-type agents are detoxified exclusively in the liver. The rate of hepatic metabolism is fastest for prilocaine but similar for lidocaine, mepivacaine, bupivacaine, and etidocaine.

SPECIFIC AGENTS

Cocaine

Cocaine, an ester, is active topically and has the ability to cause vasoconstriction by blocking reuptake of norepinephrine at sympathetic nerve endings. Its use is limited to anesthetizing the mucous membrane of the upper airway by topical application.

Procaine

Procaine is also an ester. Hydrolysis of procaine in the body yields para-aminobenzoic acid, which is known to interfere with the bacteriostatic action of sulfonamides. The agent is not active topically. A 0.25% or 0.5% solution is adequate for local infiltration or extensive field blocks, but a 1% or 2% solution is required for nerve blocks. Depending on the concentration used, its duration of action is anywhere from 30 minutes to 1 hour. It is a relatively safe agent; as much as 15 mg/kg can be given without signs of systemic toxicity.

Chloroprocaine

Chloroprocaine is a chlorinated derivative of procaine. The two agents have similar properties, but chloroprocaine is more potent. It is also more rapidly hydrolyzed and has a shorter duration of action than the parent compound. The maximal safe dose is

15 mg/kg. (There have been reports of neurotoxicity following intrathecal injection of chloroprocaine. Although toxicity may have been due to the presence of sodium bisulfite preservative and the low pH of the solution and not to the drug itself, choloroprocaine is not recommended for spinal anesthesia.)

Tetracaine

Tetracaine, another ester, is 10 times as potent as procaine. A dose of over 1.5 mg/kg is toxic. This agent is used almost exclusively for spinal anesthesia. A 1% solution is usually mixed with an equal volume of 10% dextrose to make a 0.5% hyperbaric solution (a solution with specific gravity higher than that of cerebrospinal fluid). Since tetracaine is hydrolyzed four times more slowly than procaine, its duration of action is up to 3 hours; this can be increased even further with the addition of a vasoconstrictor.

Lidocaine

Lidocaine, an amide, is by far a better agent than procaine. The advantages are rapid onset, more intense anesthesia, and a longer duration of action. Onset of action can be hastened and intensity of anesthesia increased even further by the use of carbonated lidocaine in place of lidocaine hydrochloride. Unlike procaine, lidocaine is also active topically. Normally a 0.5% solution is used for local infiltration, a 1% or 2% solution for nerve blocks, a 1.5% or 2% solution for epidural anesthesia, and a 5% solution for spinal anesthesia. Epinephrine may be added to increase its duration of action. In addition, 2% and 4% syrup are available for use as a mouthwash or gargle, 4% solution and 10% aerosol for topical anesthesia of the trachea, and 2% jelly and 5% ointment for lubrication of endotracheal tubes.

Lidocaine is a safe and effective local anesthetic. It is the most popular agent in current practice. In order to avoid systemic toxicity, its dose should be limited to 7 mg/kg with epinephrine or 5 mg/kg without.

Dibucaine

Dibucaine, also an amide, is a potent but toxic agent. Its action is slow in onset but lasts 2–3 hours. Prepared as a 0.5% solution, it is used almost exclusively for spinal anesthesia. Systemic toxicity is seen when the dose exceeds 1.5 mg/kg.

Prilocaine

The action of prilocaine, another amide, is somewhat similar to that of lidocaine, but it is less toxic. As much as 9 mg/kg with epinephrine or 6 mg/kg without epinephrine is tolerated by most subjects. However prilocaine can cause the formation of methemoglobin, a product of oxidation of the ferrous iron of normal hemoglobin to the ferric state by toluidine, a metabolite of prilocaine. Methemoglobin does not have the ability to carry oxygen, and signs of severe methemoglobinemia are those of hypoxemia. A patient who develops clinical signs related to methemoglobinemia should be treated with oxygen by mask, and methylene blue, 1–2 mg/kg, should be given intravenously. Methylene blue is a reducing agent capable of converting methemoglobin to normal hemoglobin.

Mepivacaine

Pharmacologically mepivacaine, also an amide, resembles lidocaine except that its duration of action is somewhat longer. A 1% solution is suitable for local infiltration, but a 1.5% solution is required for major nerve blocks and a 1.5% or 2% solution for epidural anesthesia. A dose of over 5 mg/kg, with or without epinephrine, is toxic.

Bupivacaine

Bupivacaine is structurally very similar to mepivacaine, but it is more potent and has a much longer duration of action (3–5 hours, depending on the site). Onset of action and uptake into the bloodstream are equally slow. Addition of epinephrine does little to increase its duration of action. A 0.25% solution is suitable for local infiltration; a 0.5% solution should be used for major nerve blocks; and both are adequate for epidural anesthesia. For spinal anesthesia the hyperbaric 0.75% solution in 8.25% dextrose in water should be used. Bupivacaine is a relatively toxic agent; a 0.75% solution for epidural anesthesia (not the hyperbaric solution for spinal anesthesia) has been withdrawn from the market. The total dose should be limited to 3 mg/kg, with or without epinephrine.

Etidocaine

Though etidocaine is related to lidocaine structurally, it is similar to bupivacaine in pharmacologic action but is less toxic. A dose of 6 mg/kg with epinephrine or 4 mg/kg without is tolerated well.

The Anesthetic Machine and Accessories

The function of the anesthetic machine (also called the gas machine) is to deliver a safe anesthetic mixture to the anesthetic circuit from which it can be inhaled by the patient. All modern machines have evolved from the continuous-flow Boyle's apparatus. In newer models mechanical ventilators and monitors are integrated with the basic unit. This chapter is dedicated to a description of the basic components and built-in safety features of the standard gas machine. Discussions of anesthetic circuits, ventilators, and monitors are presented in Chapters 8, 9, and 14, respectively.

BASIC COMPONENTS

Taken in the direction of gas flow, the basic components of an anesthetic machine are arranged in the following sequence (Fig. 7–1):

1. Source of oxygen, nitrous oxide, and other anesthetic gases (e.g., carbon dioxide, air)
2. Pressure gauges
3. Pressure regulators (pressure-reducing valves)
4. Flowmeters
5. One or more vaporizers for volatile agents
6. Common gas outlet
7. Oxygen flush control

Source of Anesthetic Gases

All anesthetic machines have duplicate supplies of both oxygen and nitrous oxide: either two cylinders of each gas or a supply of oxygen and nitrous oxide by pipelines and a spare supply of

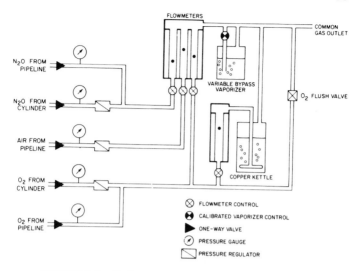

FIGURE 7–1. Basic components of the anesthetic machine.

oxygen and nitrous oxide by cylinder. These gas supplies are harnessed to the gas inlets of the machine by noninterchangeable safety systems so that a gas supply cannot be mistakenly connected to the wrong inlet (see "Safety Features" below). Within these inlets are one-way valves to prevent leakage of gases through an open inlet. Some machines are also equipped with noninterchangeable safety harnesses for the supply of air, carbon dioxide, and other anesthetic gases.

Pressure Gauges

Built into the anesthetic machine are pressure gauges for monitoring the pressure of gas supplies. Oxygen and nitrous oxide are supplied through pipelines at a constant pressure of 50 pounds per square inch (ppsi), but oxygen, nitrous oxide, and other gases are also supplied in cylinders at much higher pressures.

Oxygen is compressed to approximately 2000 ppsi in a full cylinder. At this pressure and at room temperature, compressed oxygen remains in the gaseous state. As the cylinder empties, pressure within it falls progressively, and the pressure registered is directly proportional to the amount of oxygen remaining in the cylinder. For example, a pressure of 1000 ppsi indicates that the cylinder is half full.

Nitrous oxide, on the other hand, is compressed to only about 750 ppsi in a full cylinder. At this pressure and at room temperature, compressed nitrous oxide is in the liquid state. The pressure registered on the pressure gauge in this instance is the vapor pressure of nitrous oxide at room temperature. As nitrous oxide vapor leaves the cylinder, more liquefied nitrous oxide evaporates to take its place; this vapor pressure does not fall as long as there is liquid nitrous oxide in the cylinder. When all the liquid nitrous oxide has evaporated, pressure in the cylinder falls rapidly as it empties. Therefore pressure in the nitrous oxide cylinder bears no relationship to the amount of liquid nitrous oxide in the cylinder. This is also true for carbon dioxide, which is normally compressed to 840 ppsi. The only method of determining the quantity of nitrous oxide or carbon dioxide remaining in a cylinder is to compare its weight with that of a full tank.

Pressure Regulators

The pressure of oxygen and nitrous oxide supplied by cylinders must be reduced to a lower and constant working pressure suitable for use in the anesthetic machine (40–50 ppsi). This is accomplished by means of pressure regulators (pressure-reducing valves). A pressure regulator is also necessary for air and carbon dioxide. Pressure regulators work on the simple principle that high pressure applied to a small area can be balanced by low pressure applied to a large area. In this manner a high-pressure inflow is transformed to a low-pressure outflow. In some anesthetic machines, the 50 ppsi pressure of oxygen and nitrous oxide from pipelines and the reduced pressure (40–50 ppsi) of oxygen and nitrous oxide from cylinders are further reduced to 16 ppsi by a *second-stage pressure regulator* before these gases are directed to the flowmeters.

Flowmeters

Flowmeters are tapered glass tubes (Thorpe tubes) calibrated individually for oxygen, nitrous oxide, and other gases. These tubes are mounted vertically and in parallel in a protective casing. The inflow into the flowmeters is regulated by controls situated at the lower end of the flowmeter assembly, and gas flows are indicated by floats in the center of these tubes. When the controls are shut off, the floats settle to the lower and narrower end of the flowmeter tubes. When the controls are turned on, the floats rise in the tubes according to the magnitude of the gas flows. Gas flows should be read from the upper edge of elongated floats and from the equator of spherical floats (Fig. 7–2). After passing through their respective flowmeters, anesthetic gases mix to form the fresh gas mixture before flowing downstream.

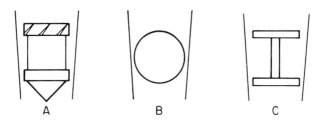

FIGURE 7–2. Types of flowmeter floats: elongated, *A* and *C*, and spherical, *B*.

Vaporizers

Vaporizers are devices designed to dispense a measured amount of volatile agent (halothane, enflurane, or isoflurane) into the fresh gas mixture. Almost all of those in use today are of the variable-bypass type (also called concentration-calibrated vaporizers). However devices with a measured flow illustrate the function of vaporizers more vividly and are described first.

The *copper kettle* is a prototype of all measured-flow vaporizers. It is supplied with its own measured flow of oxygen (Fig. 7–3*A*). As oxygen flows through the vaporizer, it becomes fully saturated

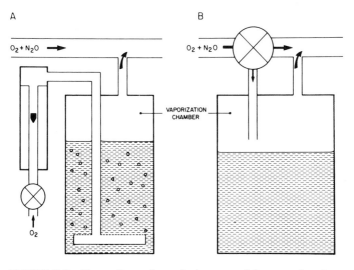

FIGURE 7–3.   Types of vaporizers. *A*, A measured-flow vaporizer (e.g., the copper kettle). *B*, A variable-bypass vaporizer (e.g., the Fluotec).

with the vapor of the volatile anesthetic. When this vapor-laden oxygen joins the fresh gas mixture, the concentration of anesthetic vapor in the mixture can be expressed as

$$\text{Concentration of vapor in anesthetic mixture} = \frac{\text{Volume of vapor}}{\text{Total volume of mixture}}$$

Since the volume of vapor is directly related to the flow of oxygen through the vaporizer, anesthetic concentration changes according to this flow.

In addition to the flow of oxygen through the vaporizer, there is one other factor that affects the vapor output of the vaporizer: cooling through loss of latent heat of vaporization. (Latent heat of vaporization may be defined as the amount of energy removed by molecules on leaving the liquid phase to enter the gaseous phase.) Although heat is absorbed from its surroundings, the temperature of the liquid anesthetic falls, with time, as it evaporates. Since vaporization is less vigorous when the liquid is cold, the volume of vapor carried by a constant flow of oxygen through the kettle is smaller at lower temperatures. That is, concentration of vapor in the anesthetic mixture falls as the liquid anesthetic cools. (The vigor of vaporization can be expressed as vapor pressure. The relationship between vapor pressure and temperature for volatile anesthetics is illustrated in Fig. 7–4). Therefore it is necessary

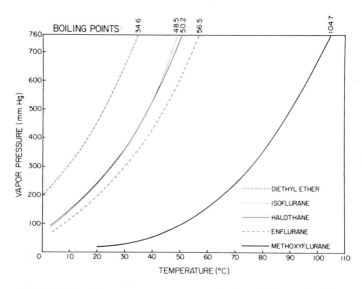

FIGURE 7–4. The vapor-pressure curves of ether, isoflurane, halothane, enflurane, and methoxyflurane.

to increase continually the flow of oxygen through the copper kettle in order to maintain a constant anesthetic vapor concentration as the liquid anesthetic cools.

The *variable-bypass vaporizer* does not have its own oxygen supply (see Fig. 7–3*B*). When such a device is switched on, a fraction of the fresh gas mixture is diverted through the vaporization chamber and becomes saturated with vapor. Subsequently this fraction rejoins the main flow downstream to yield the anesthetic mixture. The anesthetic concentration in this mixture can be calculated as for the copper kettle and is calibrated directly on the control dial. It is equipped with a temperature-sensitive mechanism that increases automatically the fraction of gas flow through the vaporization chamber as the temperature of the liquid anesthetic falls. Thus the output of anesthetic vapor remains constant, despite cooling of the vaporizer and its content. These vaporizers are calibrated individually for specific volatile agents. Filling a vaporizer with the wrong agent can cause serious overdose.

Common Gas Outlet

Beyond the vaporizer, the anesthetic mixture is directed by internal circuits to leave the anesthetic machine at the common gas outlet. This fresh gas outlet has a standard 22-mm outer diameter and a 15-mm inner diameter. From this common gas outlet, the anesthetic mixture flows to the anesthetic circuit.

Oxygen Flush Control

All anesthetic machines are equipped with an emergency oxygen flush valve. The control of this valve is usually situated close to the common gas outlet. Irrespective of flowmeter and vaporizer settings, activation of this demand valve will deliver pure oxygen at a flow of 35–75 L/min via a bypass to the common gas outlet. In older models, this control can be locked in the ON position. Using this locking feature is inadvisable because it runs the risk of allowing high pressures to build up in the anesthetic circuit and in the patient's airway. The oxygen flush valve in all modern machines is activated only on demand.

SAFETY FEATURES

In order to ensure that a safe anesthetic mixture is delivered to the patient and to avoid abuse, standards organizations, government agencies, and the industry have established safety specifications for the design of anesthetic machines and their accessories. Since there are national, regional, and institutional differences in these standards, the student is advised to become familiar with local practice. These safeguards are by no means foolproof, but in general the following features are recommended:

1. Color codes for all equipment containing or delivering medical gases and volatile anesthetics
2. Medical gas cylinders built and tested to specifications and equipped with the pin-index safety system and a safety pressure-relief valve
3. Noninterchangeable safety systems to connect medical gas pipelines to the anesthetic machine
4. A downstream position for the oxygen flowmeter in the flowmeter assembly and a unique oxygen flowmeter control
5. A safety system to fill agent-specific vaporizers
6. Mutually exclusive vaporizer controls
7. A back-pressure check valve, oxygen failure safety valve, oxygen failure alarm, minimum oxygen flow-ratio controller, and oxygen analyzer with alarm.

Color Codes

Color codes for equipment containing or delivering medical gases are designed to minimize accidental confusion sometimes encountered in the use of such equipment. In all English-speaking countries except the United States, the international code is used: white for oxygen, white and black for air, gray for carbon dioxide, black for nitrogen, blue for nitrous oxide, and brown for helium. In the United States, green replaces white for oxygen and yellow replaces white and black for air; otherwise the code is the same for the other gases mentioned. All pipelines, gas cylinders, pressure gauges, and flowmeters and their controls should be appropriately color coded.

Volatile agents are coded according to one universally accepted standard: red for halothane, orange for enflurane, purple for isoflurane, and brown for methoxyflurane. This code should be used to differentiate the containers of these agents and agent-specific vaporizers.

Medical Gas Cylinders

The oxygen and nitrous oxide cylinders most commonly mounted on anesthetic machines are size E cylinders made of steel or its chromium-molybdenum alloy. All cylinders in use are tested every 5–10 years; they should withstand a pressure two-thirds higher than the maximum allowable working pressure. However the pressure in a full cylinder containing liquefied or flammable gases should not exceed the working pressure at room temperature, and the pressure in a full cylinder containing nonliquefied and nonflammable gases should not exceed the working pressure by more than 10%. All information concerning the manufacturing and testing of such a cylinder is engraved on its shoulder (Fig. 7–5A, B). A large label bearing the chemical or common name of its contents is affixed to its body, and a tag indicating whether the cylinder is full or empty is attached to its neck (Fig. 7–5C). When the cylinder is in use, the FULL section of the tag should be removed; when the cylinder is empty, the IN USE section should be removed.

At the upper end of the cylinder, there is an elongated block in which resides the cylinder valve (Fig. 7–6). Gas flow through the outlet port of this valve is controlled by turning the valve stem counterclockwise with a wrench. Two safety features are built into this valve block: the pin-index safety system and the safety pressure-relief valve.

Pin-Index Safety System. Gas cylinders are secured to the anesthetic machine by yokes. The pin-index safety system is designed to prevent the attachment of a cylinder to the wrong inlet

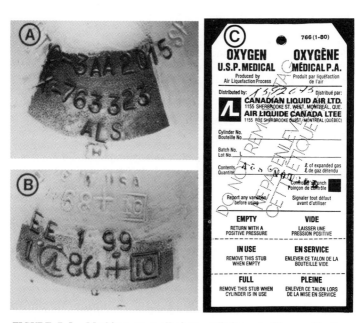

FIGURE 7–5. Markings on medical gas cylinders. *A*, The specification number of the cylinder is *3AA*; *2015* is the service pressure in ppsi; *X-763323* is the serial number; and *ALS* identifies the owner. *B*, The marking *EE19.9* is the elastic expansion in ml at 3360 ppsi; *1–80* is the retest date; the symbol between *1* and *80* identifies the testing facility; and *+10* indicates that 10% overfill is allowable. *C*, The label attached to the neck of the cylinder.

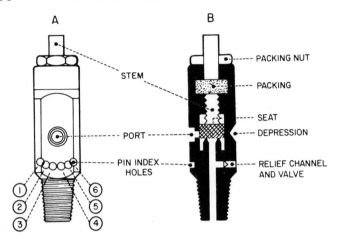

FIGURE 7–6. The cylinder valve. *A*, Frontal view illustrating the loci of the pin-index holes. *B*, Cross section illustrating the valve mechanism and the safety pressure relief valve.

on the anesthetic machine (e.g., a nitrous oxide cylinder to the oxygen inlet). This is achieved by the presence of two holes just below the exit port of the valve block. These holes are matched by two corresponding pins on the yoke. Each of these holes, with the corresponding pin, occupies one of six loci describing an arc (see Fig. 7–6A). Two exclusive loci of holes and pins have been assigned to each gas. If a cylinder is attached to the wrong yoke, the unmatched position of pins and holes will prevent proper alignment of the outlet port of the cylinder and the inlet port of the anesthetic machine. The loci allocated for oxygen are 2 and 5; those for nitrous oxide are 3 and 5; those for air are 1 and 5.

Safety Pressure-Relief Valve. The safety pressure-relief valve (see Fig. 7–6B) is designed to prevent rupture of the cylinder should the pressure within rise rapidly above working pressure (e.g., during a fire). Usually one of three valve mechanisms is employed: a metal disk that ruptures at high pressure, an alloy that has a relatively low melting point (e.g., Wood's metal), or a spring-loaded one-way valve that yields to high pressure.

Noninterchangeable Pipeline Connections

Pipelines delivering compressed gases are also attached to the anesthetic machine by noninterchangeable connections. Two such systems exist: the diameter-index safety system and the quick-mount system.

The *diameter-index safety system* is illustrated in Figure 7–7A.

It consists of a female component having two concentric bores (M and N) that will mate with a corresponding male component having two concentric diameters (M' and N'). The diameters of M and N and those of M' and N' are specific for each gas. As diameters M and M' increase, those of N and N' decrease. In this manner, the female component designed for a specific gas is absolutely incompatible with the male component of all other gases.

With the diameter-index safety system, time and tools are required for making connections and disconnections. The *quick-mount system*, on the other hand, allows rapid connection and disconnection without special tools. There is more than one type of quick-mount system. Figure 7–7*B* illustrates one type in which the index skirt of the male component must fit the index groove of the female counterpart. The two components are held together by a spring-loaded catch (the pawl) engaging the retaining groove. Turning the sleeve clockwise will release this catch and allow rapid disconnection. In another type, the female component has concentric bores that match the concentric diameters of the corresponding male component. Noninterchangeability is ensured in a manner similar to that of the diameter-index safety system. These two components are held together by plunging the male element into the female element and locking them together with a counterclockwise twist.

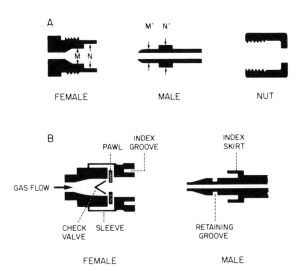

FIGURE 7–7. Non-interchangeable pipeline connections. *A*, The diameter-index safety system. *B*, One type of quick-mount system.

Oxygen Flowmeter and Its Control

In order to minimize the possibility of delivering a hypoxic gas mixture due to leaks, all anesthetic machines manufactured in North America since 1974 have their oxygen flowmeter located downstream of all other flowmeters in the flowmeter assembly. If the oxygen flowmeter were mounted in the upstream position, oxygen could escape through cracks in all flowmeters (see Fig. 7–8A). This can result in the delivery of a hypoxic gas mixture if nitrous oxide is also turned on. With the oxygen flowmeter mounted downstream, oxygen is lost only if there is a leak in its own flowmeter tube (Fig. 7–8B), so the chance of a hypoxic mixture being delivered is reduced.

In English-speaking countries other than the United States and Canada, the oxygen flowmeter is left in the upstream position but oxygen flows in its own conduit to enter the mainstream at a point distal to all other flowmeters (Fig. 7–8C). This arrangement has the same margin of safety as that used in North America.

Much effort has also been put into the design of the oxygen flowmeter control. To allow it to be distinguishable from others under all lighting conditions, certain features are recommended: it should be coded by color, have the chemical formula O_2 affixed to its face, have a profile unique to sight and to touch, and be the most accessible of all the flowmeter controls.

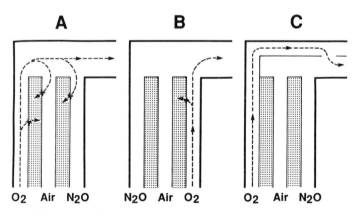

A   **B**   **C**

O_2 Air N_2O N_2O Air O_2 O_2 Air N_2O

FIGURE 7–8. Position of oxygen flowmeter. If it is mounted upstream, *A*, a leak in any of the flowmeters can result in the delivery of a hypoxic gas mixture. If it is mounted downstream, *B*, a hypoxic gas mixture is delivered only when the leak is in the oxygen flowmeter itself. If the oxygen flowmeter is upstream but oxygen is allowed to flow in its own conduit to a point distal to all other flowmeters, *C*, the risk of oxygen leak is the same as that in *B*.

Agent-Specific Filling System for Vaporizers

All modern variable-bypass vaporizers are agent specific. Accidental filling of a vaporizer with the wrong agent not only can cause serious misunderstandings but also can lead to fatal overdose. The agent-specific filling system for vaporizers is designed to avoid such accidents.

The filling port of a vaporizer without this system is simply a funnel, but that of a vaporizer with this system is housed in a block that will accept only the tip of a spout with an index groove carved into its side (Fig. 7–9). At the other end of the spout, the bottle cap also has grooves at its side so that it will fit only containers that have a collar with matching ridges. The vaporizer, the spout, and the bottle are also color coded for the agent.

Exclusive Vaporizer Control

In order to prevent more than one vaporizer from being switched on simultaneously, vaporizer controls should be exclusive. In older models, the intended agent has to be selected on a separate control first. Only then can the control of the vaporizer containing that agent be switched on. No amount of tampering will allow the control of a second vaporizer to be turned on simultaneously. In

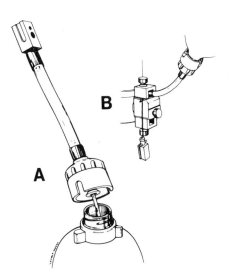

FIGURE 7–9.   Filling spout used in agent-specific filling system for vaporizers. *A*, Grooves in cap and in block allow connection only to appropriate containers. *B*, The connected spout.

current models, the controls of these vaporizers are mutually exclusive. That is, once the control of one vaporizer is switched on, the controls of the others are automatically locked in the OFF position.

Back-Pressure Check Valve

During positive-pressure ventilation of the patient, intermittent positive pressure applied to the anesthetic circuit will travel in both anterograde and retrograde directions. Therefore back-pressure is transmitted to the vaporization chamber of the vaporizer that is in use. At the commencement of expiration, the rapid fall in back-pressure will cause a simple vaporizer (e.g., the Boyle's bottle) to discharge both at its inlet and its outlet (Fig. 7–10), thereby increasing the anesthetic output of the vaporizer. A second problem related to back-pressure is bouncing movements of flowmeter floats: a fall in the levels of the floats when positive pressure is applied and a rise to normal levels when positive pressure is removed. Interposition of a one-way check valve between the distal vaporizer and the common gas outlet eliminates these problems. (Back-pressure has no effect on the vapor output of a modern vaporizer.)

Oxygen Failure Safety Valve

The oxygen failure safety valve is a mechanical device designed to interrupt the flow of nitrous oxide and other inert gases to the anesthetic circuit before oxygen supply pressure has fallen to 25 ppsi. (Oxygen supply pressure is the pressure of oxygen in the

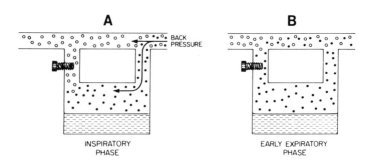

FIGURE 7–10. The effect of back-pressure on a simple variable-bypass vaporizer. During controlled ventilation, pressurization of the vaporizer during inspiration, *A*, can lead to the discharge of vapor at both the inlet and the outlet of the vaporizer in the early expiratory phase, *B*. The fresh gas is represented by open dots; the vapor-laden mixture, by solid dots.

pipeline or of oxygen from the cylinder after it has gone through the first-stage pressure regulator. It is 40–50 ppsi.) This interruption of inert gas flow is achieved either by shutting off the supply of all gases or by venting these gases into the atmosphere at a point distal to the flowmeters. It must be stressed that this safety valve ensures only that no hypoxic gas mixture is delivered to the anesthetic circuit when oxygen supply fails. It *does not protect* against failure in oxygen supply, *nor does it prevent* the delivery of a hypoxic gas mixture due to leaks in the flowmeter assembly or at a point distal to this assembly. When *oxygen supply pressure is normal*, it is possible to turn on the flow of nitrous oxide or other inert gases *without switching on the oxygen flow*.

Oxygen Failure Alarm

The oxygen failure alarm is an adjunct to the safety valve. As oxygen supply fails, the alarm will sound a high-pitched warning for at least 7 seconds. In some of these devices, the failing source of oxygen is used to sound the alarm, which will stop when the supply of oxygen is depleted. Stoppage of the audio signal in this instance should not be regarded as correction of the problem. In another type, the audio alarm is powered by nitrous oxide. However, if nitrous oxide is not in use, the alarm will fail to function. A third type powered by battery is also available, but will not function if the battery becomes exhausted. Therefore these devices should not be regarded as foolproof.

Minimum Oxygen Flow-Ratio Controller

This is a mechanical link between the oxygen and nitrous oxide flowmeter controls. Its function is twofold: to provide a minimal flow of oxygen at 200 ml/min and maintain oxygen flow above 25% of total flow at all times. When both oxygen and nitrous oxide are in use (e.g., 2 L/min flow each), nothing will happen to nitrous oxide flow if oxygen flow is increased beyond 2 L/min. Nothing will happen to nitrous oxide flow either if oxygen flow is reduced to less than 2 L/min, as long as oxygen flow remains above 25% of total flow. But if oxygen flow is reduced to below 667 ml/min (less than 25% of total flow), then nitrous oxide flow will decrease pro rata automatically to maintain oxygen flow at 25% of total flow. When oxygen flow falls to 200 ml/min, nitrous oxide flow shuts off automatically. In the same example, oxygen flow will rise pro rata automatically if nitrous oxide flow is increased beyond 2 L/min to a point when oxygen flow is less than 25% of total flow.

Introduction of this oxygen-nitrous oxide controller represents another step to prevent dispensing hypoxic mixtures from the anesthetic machine. Again this effort is not foolproof. Since this controller links the oxygen and nitrous oxide flowmeter controls only, addition of a second inert gas (some machines are equipped with carbon dioxide, nitrogen, or helium flowmeters) can result in the delivery of hypoxic mixtures.

Oxygen Analyzer with Alarm

Besides prevention, it is equally important to be warned of the danger when a hypoxic gas mixture has been delivered. Addition of an oxygen analyzer with an alarm is a step in this direction. This device is an add-on feature in older machines but a built-in component of newer models. It emits an audible alarm and a visual signal when oxygen concentration of the gas mixture falls below 21%. If the alarm does go off, the sole means of resetting it is by increasing oxygen concentration to 21% or more.

The oxygen analyzer used for this purpose has a slow response time and becomes inaccurate if moisture condenses on the surface of its electrode (see "Galvanic Fuel Cell and Polarographic Oxygen Analyzers" in Chap. 14). Therefore locating the analyzer electrode in the expiratory limb of any anesthetic circuit is undesirable. It should be incorporated into the inspiratory limb of the circle system and be positioned at the common gas outlet when other circuits are used.

Anesthetic Circuits

The anesthetic circuit delivers the anesthetic mixture from the machine to the patient's upper airway. Common to all anesthetic circuits are the tubings, relief valve (expiratory valve), and reservoir bag. Since the lungs can be injured by high pressures built up accidentally in the circuit, a safety valve that blows off at 40 cm H_2O also should be incorporated into the system (e.g., the Norry valve).

CIRCUIT COMPONENTS

Anesthetic Tubings

Anesthetic tubings are made of antistatic black rubber or light-weight plastic. They form a low-resistance conduit through which the anesthetic mixture is delivered to the patient's upper airway, and they act as a reservoir in which fresh anesthetic mixture is stored during expiration. Tubing for adult circuits has a 22-mm inner diameter and that for pediatric circuits, a 15-mm inner diameter.

Relief Valve

In current anesthetic practice the rate at which fresh gas is added to the circuit is higher than the rate of uptake by the patient. Therefore it is necessary to include a relief valve (also called *expiratory valve*) in the circuit to vent excess gas to the atmosphere or to a scavenging system. A prototype relief valve is illustrated in Figure 8–1A. The valve is shut by turning the control clockwise; it is opened by turning the control in the other direction. When the valve is shut, compression of the spring pushes the valve disk tight against its seat, so that no gas can escape. When the valve is open, the spring is only lightly compressed; excess gas escapes through the vent by unseating the valve disk.

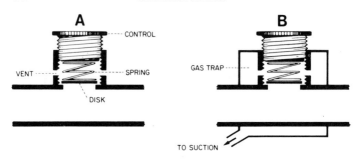

FIGURE 8–1. The relief valve (expiratory valve). *A*, A simple relief valve. *B*, A scavenging device.

Some relief valves are built within a gas trap (see Fig. 8–1*B*) from which the overflow is removed by suction or is directed to the outflow of the central ventilation system. These are called *scavenging devices;* they are designed to reduce pollution of the operating room atmosphere.

The setting of the relief valve varies according to the mode of ventilation. During spontaneous ventilation the valve should be set fully open so that excess gas can vent at a low pressure during expiration. During manual ventilation the valve should be set partially closed so that pressure applied to the reservoir bag and transmitted to the circuit can inflate the patient's lungs until the opening pressure of the valve is reached, when some of the gas mixture is vented. During mechanical ventilation the valve should be shut and excess gas should be allowed to overflow through the ventilator. The relief valve should *never* be completely shut except during mechanical ventilation.

Reservoir Bag

The function of the reservoir bag is exactly as its name implies. During inspiration, inspiratory flow varies. It is zero at the beginning of inspiration; it rises to approximately 30 L/min at its peak; and it settles back to zero at the end of inspiration. Fresh gas flow from the anesthetic machine, on the other hand, is constant and is not set nearly as high as peak inspiratory flow. Therefore there are moments during inspiration when a large discrepancy between fresh gas flow and inspiratory flow exists. This shortfall is drawn from the reservoir bag as required. In addition, the reservoir bag also serves as a monitor of the patient's ventilatory function during spontaneous ventilation and provides a means by which the patient's lungs can be ventilated manually.

TYPE OF CIRCUITS

In the past it has been popular to classify anesthetic circuits into open, semiopen, semiclosed, and closed systems and the respective terms were used ambiguously. Classifying circuits as rebreathing and non-rebreathing systems is equally unsatisfactory because some degree of rebreathing occurs with all commonly used circuits. In this chapter circuits are identified by their common names. The most popular circuits in current use are the anesthetic circle, the Magill circuit, the modified T-piece, and the Bain circuit. For completeness, the Waters to-and-fro system and circuits employing non-rebreathing valves are also mentioned.

The Circle System

The anesthetic circle is the most popular circuit in use in North America. When the fresh gas flow added to the circle is low, rebreathing of expired gas is marked, but carbon dioxide in the expired gas is removed by a soda lime or a baralyme canister incorporated into the circuit.

Soda lime comes in 4- to 8-mesh granules hardened with a small amount of silicates (4-mesh has 16 quarter-inch openings psi; 8-mesh has 64 eighth-inch openings psi). The granules are composed of 4% sodium hydroxide, 1% potassium hydroxide, 76–81% calcium hydroxide, 14–19% moisture, and a dye indicator. The reactions involved in carbon dioxide absorption are as follows:

$$CO_2 + H_2O \rightarrow H_2CO_3$$

$$2\ NaOH + H_2CO_3 \rightarrow Na_2CO_3 + 2\ H_2O$$

$$Ca(OH)_2 + H_2CO_3 \rightarrow CaCO_3 + 2\ H_2O$$

These reactions generate heat. Although water is also generated, the presence of moisture is essential to initiate these reactions. A change in the color of the pH-sensitive dye indicator is a sign of exhaustion of the absorbent. (The exact color change varies with the brand.)

Baralyme is 20% barium hydroxide octahydrate and 80% calcium hydroxide. It also comes in 4-mesh or 8-mesh granules. Carbon dioxide reacts with barium hydroxide octahydrate directly according to the equation

$$Ba(OH)_2 \cdot 8\ H_2O + CO_2 \rightarrow BaCO_3 + 9\ H_2O$$

The most popular arrangement of the circle is illustrated in Figure 8–2. There are two relief valves in the circle: one near the patient on the Y-piece and one close to the reservoir bag. In spontaneous ventilation, overflow occurs during the second half of expiration. This should be allowed to take place at the relief valve near the

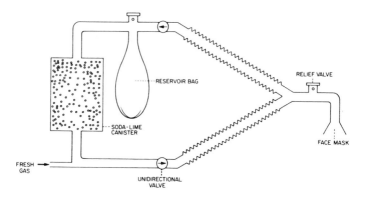

FIGURE 8–2. The circle system.

patient to vent expired gas. In manual ventilation, overflow occurs during inspiration. To minimize escape of fresh gas through the valve near the patient, this valve should be shut and overflow allowed to take place at the one close to the reservoir bag. The circle system has these advantages over other circuits:

1. Economy of low fresh gas flow
2. Partial warming and humidification of the inspired mixture
3. Little overflow of excess gas and less pollution of the operating room atmosphere
4. Reduced fire hazard when flammable agents are used.

A major disadvantage of the system is its high resistance, which is less than ideal for small children. Resistance can be reduced by removing the unidirectional valves and using a circulator instead to direct gas flow.

Most anesthesiologists using the circle system choose a fresh gas flow of 2–3 L/min. With this magnitude of fresh gas flow, rebreathing is only partial. The technique is safe so long as the fresh gas mixture contains at least 25% oxygen. Yet to maximize the advantages of the anesthetic circle requires reduction of fresh gas flow to around 200 ml/min of 100% oxygen, just enough to meet the basal metabolic rate. At this very low flow, rebreathing is maximal. This closed-circuit technique carries certain risks. Owing to dilution of fresh gas by exhaled gases, there is always a huge discrepancy between oxygen concentration of the fresh gas (which is 100%) and that of the mixture in the inspiratory limb of the circle. Large changes in vaporizer settings are required to bring about small changes in anesthetic concentration of the inspired mixture, and minor incompetence of unidirectional valves can cause dangerous accumulation of carbon dioxide in the circuit.

Oxygen concentration and carbon dioxide tension of inspired and expired gases should be monitored at the airway when low flow technique is practiced.

Magill Circuit

The arrangement of the Magill circuit (also called the Mapleson A circuit) is illustrated in Figure 8–3. Since carbon dioxide absorption is not employed, adequate flow of fresh gas is required to purge the circuit of expired gas. In order to minimize rebreathing, fresh gas flow equal to the patient's minute ventilatory volume (approximately 100 ml/kg body weight) is sufficient during spontaneous ventilation. However a very high gas flow is required to minimize rebreathing during controlled ventilation, a feature that makes this circuit impractical for this purpose.

Ayre's T-piece

There are many modifications of the original Ayre's T-piece; the most popular is the Jackson-Rees version (see Fig. 8–3). (This circuit is called the Mapleson E circuit if the reservoir bag is omitted). Being valveless, it offers little resistance to gas flow; this feature makes it the most popular pediatric circuit in use today. During spontaneous ventilation overflow from the system is allowed to escape through the open end of the reservoir bag; during manual ventilation the open end of the reservoir bag is occluded as the bag is compressed; and during mechanical ventilation this bag is replaced by the bellows of the mechanical ventilator. The modified T-piece is not as efficient as the Magill circuit

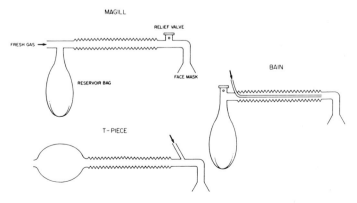

FIGURE 8–3. The Magill circuit, the T-piece, and the Bain circuit.

in eliminating expired gas during spontaneous ventilation: A fresh gas flow 2.5–3 times the patient's minute volume is required to prevent rebreathing. On the other hand, it is more efficient than the Magill circuit during controlled ventilation and fresh gas flows required to maintain normocapnia in the patient are

1. For patients weighing 10–30 kg: 100 ml/kg body weight plus 1000 ml

2. For patients weighing more than 30 kg: 50 ml/kg body weight plus 2000 ml

Bain Circuit

The Bain circuit (see Fig. 8–3) is made of lightweight plastic and is a modification of the Mapleson D circuit. Its extra length allows the anesthetic machine to be positioned well away from the field of operation, which has made it popular in anesthesia for head and neck surgery. During spontaneous ventilation a fresh gas flow of 100–150 ml/kg body weight is required to minimize rebreathing. Unlike the Magill circuit, it is more efficient during controlled than during spontaneous ventilation. A fresh gas flow of 70 ml/kg body weight is sufficient to maintain normocapnia.

Waters to-and-fro Circuit

The Waters to-and-fro circuit (Fig. 8–4) is a carbon dioxide absorption system that offers low resistance to gas flow yet has all the advantages of the circle system. Being located close to the patient's head, the Waters canister is cumbersome and can shed irritant alkaline dust into the airway. Its popularity is waning.

Circuit with Non-rebreathing Valves

A non-rebreathing valve (e.g., Ambu, Fink, Reuben, Stephen-Slater) is one that directs fresh gas mixture to the patient during

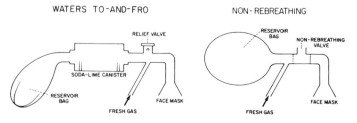

FIGURE 8–4. The Waters to-and-fro circuit and a circuit with non-rebreathing valve.

inspiration and expired mixture to the atmosphere during expiration. A prototype circuit is illustrated in Figure 8–4. During spontaneous ventilation fresh gas flow should be adjusted so that the reservoir bag is between half and three-fourths full at the end of expiration. During controlled ventilation fresh gas flow should equal the patient's minute volume. Unfortunately many of these valves have a significant apparatus dead space; some can become incompetent with use; others can stick when wet; and all are difficult to clean and sterilize. These circuits are not popular except in cardiopulmonary resuscitation (see "Advanced Life Support" in Chap. 22).

Mechanical Ventilators

Mechanical ventilators are devices that generate positive pressure rhythmically to inflate the lungs during artificial ventilation. All ventilators have the following functions: (1) to inflate the lungs during inspiration, (2) to change over from inspiration to expiration, (3) to deflate the lungs during expiration, and (4) to change over from expiration to inspiration. Ideally all ventilators should also be equipped with these devices: a gauge to monitor pressure in the circuit, a low-pressure alarm, a pressure-limiting device to protect the lungs from barotrauma, and a spirometer to measure ventilatory volumes.

PHASES OF VENTILATION

Inspiratory Phase

All mechanical ventilators are driven either by compressed gas or by electric motor. When the generated pressure is applied to the upper airway, flow of air into the lungs and the volume of inflation are determined by these equations:

$$\text{Flow} = \frac{\text{Airway-alveolar pressure gradient}}{\text{Airway resistance}}$$

$$\text{Volume} = \text{Increase in alveolar pressure} \times \text{Compliance}$$

The magnitude of positive pressure a ventilator generates can be low or very high. When it is low but constant, the *pressure* transmitted to the upper airway is *constant* throughout inspiration (see Fig. 9–1A). Flow into the lungs is high initially but falls exponentially to zero at the end of inspiration (see Fig. 9–1B). A ventilator producing this type of pressure is called a *constant-pressure generator.*

When the generated pressure is very high, this pressure is usually applied to the airway gradually so that airway pressure increases throughout inspiration (see Fig. 9–1C). *Flow* into the lungs,

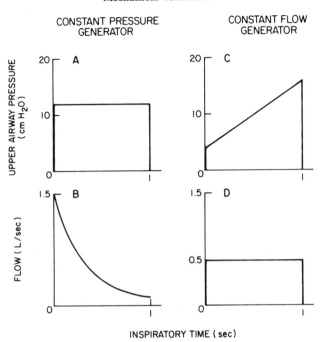

CONSTANT PRESSURE GENERATOR

CONSTANT FLOW GENERATOR

INSPIRATORY TIME (sec)

FIGURE 9–1. The pressure and flow wave forms of a constant-pressure generator and a constant-flow generator.

however, is *constant* (see Fig. 9–1*D*). A ventilator producing this type of air flow is called a *constant-flow generator.*

Changes in compliance or airway resistance of the lungs will affect the performance of these ventilators in different ways. A constant-pressure generator delivering a set volume to normal lungs will have difficulty delivering this same volume when compliance falls, airway resistance increases, or when both happen simultaneously. A constant-flow generator, on the other hand, is a powerful machine. It delivers the same volume at the expense of higher airway pressure, even when compliance and airway resistance deteriorate.

When volume delivered is the sole criterion, performance of a constant-pressure generator is affected by changes in lung characteristics, whereas that of a constant-flow generator is not. The right type of ventilator should be chosen to match the patient's lung characteristics. In the operating room, use of a constant-pressure generator is not unreasonable because most anesthetized patients have stable lung characteristics. In critically ill patients whose pulmonary compliance and airway resistance can change from moment to moment, only a constant-flow generator can deliver a constant volume of ventilation.

Changeover from Inspiration to Expiration

For a ventilator to function effectively, it must stop inflation periodically to allow the lungs to deflate. There are four types of changeover mechanism: volume cycling, time cycling, pressure cycling, and flow cycling.

In *volume cycling,* changeover occurs after the ventilator has delivered a preset volume. Owing to the presence of small leaks and distensibility of delivery tubings, this volume is always larger than that received by the patient. Nevertheless it is a common design used in many ventilators.

Time cycling is equally popular, and changeover occurs after a preset inspiratory time. When time cycling is used in a constant-flow generator, changeover occurs only after a preset volume has been delivered (volume is the product of flow and time).

In *pressure cycling,* changeover occurs when pressure at the upper airway has reached a preset value. When a ventilator is pressure cycled, the volume it delivers varies according to the changing characteristics of the lungs. That is, a pressure-cycled constant-flow generator behaves as a constant-pressure generator.

In *flow cycling,* changeover occurs when inspiratory flow has fallen to a preset value. This mechanism is used only in low-pressure generators.

Expiratory Phase

During expiratory phase the lungs are allowed to deflate, usually against atmospheric pressure but in some cases against a positive end-expiratory pressure (PEEP). Use of negative pressure in the expiratory phase is now out of favor.

Changeover from Expiration to Inspiration

Ability of the ventilator to change over from expiration to inspiration is as important as that from inspiration to expiration. Although the same four changeover mechanisms can be defined, only changeover after a preset expiratory time (i.e., time cycling) is practical.

SAFETY DEVICES

Mechanical ventilation is indispensable in a modern operating room, and safeguards should be in place to monitor its function. Some of these devices are built in to the ventilator and some are added-on components. When the mechanical ventilator is an integral part of the modern anesthetic machine, these devices are integrated into the array of monitors of the machine.

Pressure Gauge and Pressure Alarm

Airway pressure should be monitored by a mechanical gauge or electronic transducing device during mechanical ventilation (see "Airway Pressure" in Chap. 14). Normally airway pressure should be near zero during end expiration (unless PEEP is applied) and should not exceed 30 cm H_2O at peak inspiration. A large increase in peak inspiratory pressure could mean an increase in airway resistance (e.g., bronchospasm or kinked endotracheal tube), a decrease in chest wall or pulmonary compliance (e.g., recovery from muscle relaxant, pneumothorax, or pulmonary congestion), or, rarely, mechanical failure of the ventilator (e.g., blocked expiratory vent). A large fall in peak inspiratory pressure during positive-pressure ventilation always means a major leak in the anesthetic circuit or even total disconnection.

Disconnection in the anesthetic circuit is a critical incident. It should be standard practice to incorporate a low-pressure alarm in the circuit to warn the operator of this danger. These alarms have two adjustable variables: alarm pressure and alarm delay. Alarm pressure is the pressure below which the alarm will be triggered; it should be set at no more than 5 cm H_2O below the patient's peak airway pressure. Alarm delay—the interval from the critical fall in peak airway pressure to sounding of the alarm— should be set at no longer than three respiratory cycles.

The correct site at which to measure pressure is open to debate. Ideally the sample line of the pressure gauge and pressure alarm should be located as close to the airway as possible; but condensation of moisture and contamination by secretions have discouraged sampling from this location. Most practitioners would accept readings from the circuit mount, at a point close to where the ventilator circuit joints the anesthetic circuit. (Capnography can also alert the operator to the danger of disconnection. See Chap. 14.)

Pressure-Limiting Device

Excess pressure generated by mechanical ventilators (particularly by constant-flow generators) can cause barotrauma to the airway and lungs (e.g., pneumothorax). Most ventilators have a pop-off valve in the internal circuit to limit the pressure that can be delivered to the upper airway. The pressure at which it pops off is either fixed by the manufacturer or is adjustable by the operator. Usually it is set at 50–70 cm H_2O.

Spirometer

The bellows of the ventilator is usually calibrated to indicate the volume of gas mixture it delivers with each breath. Owing to compression of the gas mixture, distention of anesthetic tubing, and minor leaks, the tidal volume received by the patient is always less than what is registered by the bellow. A spirometer mounted on the expiratory limb of the anesthetic circuit can give independent verification of tidal and minute volumes. Changes in ventilatory volume can raise warning to changes in lung characteristics and disconnections (see "Ventilatory Volumes" in Chap. 14).

A PRACTICAL GUIDE TO MECHANICAL VENTILATION

Pulmonary capillary blood absorbs oxygen from and excretes carbon dioxide into the alveoli. The purpose of pulmonary ventilation is to bring oxygen into and remove carbon dioxide from the alveoli. When this is done properly, not only is an adequate volume of air moving in and out of the lungs, but also the distribution of this volume to the alveoli matches their perfusion (see Chap. 10). Therefore choice of tidal volume, respiratory rate, and inspiration-expiration ratio (or inspiratory and expiratory times) is important. In addition the positive intrathoracic pressure during mechanical inflation of the lungs can impede venous return to the heart. In order to minimize this undesirable side-effect of positive-pressure ventilation, proper selection of inspiration-expiration ratio again is important.

Tidal Volume

Tidal volume delivered by mechanical ventilators can be set by adjusting the volume control or by adjusting both the inspiratory flow and inspiratory time controls. (Volume is the product of flow and time.) Tidal volume of a normal person in the awake state is approximately 7 ml/kg body weight. For reasons stated in Chapter 10, tidal volume of normal anesthetized persons should be increased by 50–100% during mechanical ventilation, to reduce ventilation-perfusion inequalities.

Respiratory Rate and Inspiration-Expiration Ratio

The respiratory rate on a mechanical ventilator can be set by the rate control alone or by adjusting both the inspiratory and expiratory time controls. Rate should be set at a normal level of 10–15 breaths per minute. In order not to impede venous return, the inspiratory phase should be as short as is practical. However delivering a set tidal volume in a short time encourages maldistribution of inspired gas and ventilation-perfusion inequalities. Experience has shown that an inspiration-expiration ratio between 1:2 and 1:1 is acceptable in normal persons.

Inspiratory Flow

Like short inspiratory time, a fast inspiratory flow encourages ventilation-perfusion inequalities. Therefore inspiratory flow should be slow. Obviously it should not be so slow that the selected tidal volume cannot be delivered in the chosen inspiratory time.

In summary, effective pulmonary ventilation can be achieved in patients who have normal lungs with the following ventilator settings: tidal volume, 10–15 ml/kg; rate, 10–15 breaths per minute; inspiration-expiration ratio, between 1:2 and 1:1; and inspiratory flow, relatively slow. Capnography is a useful aid in the fine adjustment of fresh gas flow, tidal volume, and respiratory rate and to keep end-tidal carbon dioxide tension between 35 and 40 mm Hg (see "Capnographs" in Chap. 14).

10

Effect of Anesthesia on Respiratory Function

Of the many systemic side-effects of anesthetic drugs (see Chaps. 2 through 6), none is more serious than those that affect the respiratory system. Depression of ventilation and maldistribution of pulmonary ventilation and blood flow are part and parcel of general anesthesia. Both can cause hypercapnia and hypoxemia. In addition airway resistance and pulmonary compliance are also affected. In this chapter these important complications of anesthesia are described, and their effects on elimination of carbon dioxide and oxygenation are reviewed.

ALVEOLAR VENTILATION

Normally a 70-kg man breathes 10–15 times each minute and has a tidal volume of 500 ml per breath (7 ml/kg body weight per breath). However only 70% of each tidal breath is distributed to the alveoli, where gas exchange takes place; the other 30% is wasted in ventilation of the conducting airways. Gas in these anatomic airways does not take part in gas exchange, and the space it occupies is called the "anatomic dead space." The relationship between alveolar ventilation per minute ($\dot{V}_A$) and tidal volume (V_T), dead space (V_D), and respiratory rate (RR) is represented by the following equation:

$$\dot{V}_A = (V_T - V_D) \times RR$$

A fall in tidal volume or respiratory rate or an increase in dead space will decrease alveolar ventilation.

Under the influence of inhalation anesthetics, tidal volume is smaller than normal. Usually there is also an increase in respiratory rate, which is most pronounced with halothane, less so with isoflurane, and least with enflurane. This pattern of shallow breathing is much less efficient than normal breathing. As the difference between tidal volume and anatomic dead space narrows, alveolar ventilation falls, despite an increase in respiratory rate.

Under the influence of narcotic analgesics, on the other hand, respiratory rate is reduced but tidal volume remains unchanged. This pattern of breathing is equally inefficient, and alveolar ventilation falls in proportion to the decrease in respiratory rate.

During anesthesia, alveolar ventilation is also reduced by an increase in dead space. Protruding the jaw and extending the neck will double the anatomic dead space. This increase is further exaggerated by instrument dead space in face masks, connectors, and rebreathing circuits. Although tracheal intubation halves the anatomic dead space, this decrease may not be enough to offset other added instrument dead space.

In summary, alveolar ventilation is less than normal in anesthetized patients who are breathing spontaneously. Its effect on elimination of carbon dioxide and oxygenation is discussed in later sections.

CONTROL OF BREATHING

Breathing is under the control of the respiratory center at the brain stem, respiratory muscles being its effectors. To meet widely different ventilatory demands imposed by activities of the body, the respiratory center receives many sensory inputs. They include impulses from central and peripheral chemoreceptors and those from receptors in the lungs and airways, in muscles and joints, and in systemic and pulmonary vasculature. This center is also under the direct influence of higher centers and the cerebral cortex.

The central chemoreceptors are located on the ventral surface of the medulla and are anatomically distinguishable from the respiratory center itself. They are sensitive to changes in the hydrogen ion concentration of cerebrospinal fluid. An increase in hydrogen ion concentration stimulates breathing, and a decrease inhibits it.

When arterial carbon dioxide tension ($PaCO_2$) rises above normal, carbon dioxide crosses the blood-brain barrier and reacts with cerebrospinal fluid to yield hydrogen ions:

$$CO_2 + H_2O \rightleftharpoons H_2CO_3 \rightleftharpoons H^+ + HCO_3^-$$

The action of these hydrogen ions on the central receptors stimulates breathing. Since carbon dioxide excretion is increased during hyperventilation, stimulation of breathing will return both the carbon dioxide level of arterial blood and the hydrogen ion concentration of cerebrospinal fluid toward normal; that is, $PaCO_2$ regulates breathing by its effect on hydrogen ion concentration of cerebrospinal fluid. It is the most important factor in the control of normal ventilation.

Less important are the peripheral chemoreceptors located at the bifurcation of the common carotid arteries and at the aortic arch. Breathing is stimulated via this route by hypoxemia, but this mechanism does not operate until arterial oxygen tension (PaO_2) has fallen to less than 60 mm Hg. Although these receptors are stimulated also by hypercapnia, they account for less than 20% of the normal ventilatory response to carbon dioxide. Receptors in the carotid bodies, but not those in the aortic bodies, are stimulated also by acidemia.

All anesthetics depress the sensitivity of the central and peripheral chemoreceptor reflex. That is, normal increases in ventilation in response to hypercapnia or hypoxemia are either depressed or abolished by these agents. While anesthetic levels of thiopental and inhalation agents depress the ventilatory response to both hypercapnia and hypoxemia, subanesthetic levels of inhalation agents (consistent with those found in patients in the recovery room) are enough to abolish the ventilatory response to hypoxemia. Ventilatory depressant effects of anesthetic agents are dose related and additive. Among the inhalation agents, nitrous oxide has the least depressant effect. If it is used as part of the anesthetic gas mixture, the concentration of volatile agents can be reduced: thus sparing the more potent depressant effects of volatile agents.

In short, anesthetized patients are ill-equipped to cope with hypercapnia and/or hypoxemia due to depression of the normal ventilatory control mechanism. Developing hypercapnia or hypoxemia may go unnoticed if only ventilatory volumes are monitored.

VENTILATION-PERFUSION INEQUALITIES

Ideally all alveoli should receive an equal share of inspired gas and cardiac output, but in reality some mismatch of ventilation and perfusion exists in normal persons. Regardless of whether they are erect, supine, or in the lateral decubitus position, pulmonary blood flow gravitates to dependent zones of the lungs. At the same time, alveolar ventilation is better in dependent zones. However, in terms of blood flow, dependent zones of the lungs are relatively underventilated, and nondependent zones, overventilated. In other words, dependent zones of the lungs have a low ventilation-perfusion ratio, and nondependent zones have a high ventilation-perfusion ratio. This ratio is commonly expressed as $\dot{V}/\dot{Q}$.

Blood perfusing areas of the lungs with a low $\dot{V}/\dot{Q}$ ratio does not become fully saturated with oxygen; these areas act as right-to-left shunts to cause desaturation of arterial blood. Ventilation of areas of the lungs with a high $\dot{V}/\dot{Q}$ ratio is more than what is necessary to oxygenate the small amount of blood perfusing these areas. Much of the tidal exchange to these areas is wasted (like dead space gas). The volume of this wasted ventilation constitutes the alveolar dead space.

Factors that decrease the $\dot{V}/\dot{Q}$ ratio of dependent zones increase arterial desaturation, and factors that increase the $\dot{V}/\dot{Q}$ ratio of nondependent zones increase alveolar dead space and decrease "effective alveolar ventilation." Three such factors are important in the conscious state: airway closure, functional residual capacity (FRC), and hypoxic pulmonary vasoconstriction; and two others are important in anesthetized patients: the effect of anesthesia itself and that of mechanical ventilation.

Airway Closure and Functional Residual Capacity

The membranous respiratory bronchioles are compressible. When their intraluminal pressure is less than pleural pressure, these microscopic airways collapse. Consequently their alveoli are isolated and cannot take part in tidal exchange. This phenomenon is called airway closure. The lung volume at which airway closure commences is called closing capacity. (The term "closing volume" is also used. It is the difference between closing capacity and residual volume). Airway closure takes place only in dependent zones. In young healthy adults, closing capacity is well below functional residual capacity (FRC), which is the lung volume at the end of a normal expiration; therefore no airway closure occurs during normal tidal breathing.

FRC can fall (e.g., in obese or pregnant patients), and closing capacity can increase above normal (e.g., in smokers and geriatric patients). When FRC is below closing capacity, small airways in dependent zones of the lungs close prematurely during normal tidal exchange. When these airways are closed, their alveoli cannot receive a full share of the tidal volume, so the $\dot{V}/\dot{Q}$ ratio of these dependent zones falls.

Hypoxic Pulmonary Vasoconstriction

Pulmonary vessels in regions where the alveoli are underventilated and low in oxygen content tend to constrict. As a result, blood is directed to well-ventilated alveoli. Although residual perfusion of those areas with a low $\dot{V}/\dot{Q}$ ratio persists, hypoxic pulmonary vasoconstriction is a functional protective mechanism that reduces ventilation-perfusion mismatch in both dependent and nondependent zones of the lungs.

Effects of Anesthesia

If distribution of ventilation and perfusion is not perfectly balanced in the conscious state, it is even worse during anesthesia. Following induction of anesthesia, the $\dot{V}/\dot{Q}$ ratio falls in dependent zones and increases in nondependent zones. This deterioration is qualitatively similar in all anesthetized patients, whether they are breathing spontaneously or are mechanically ventilated. Although the mechanism has not been fully explained, anesthesia is known to produce certain effects on factors that control the distribution of ventilation and perfusion:

1. A 15–20% fall in FRC is a consistent feature following induction of anesthesia. FRC may even fall below closing capacity in some anesthetized patients. When this happens, the $\dot{V}/\dot{Q}$ ratio of dependent zones falls below normal.

2. Hypoxic pulmonary vasoconstriction, a protective mechanism that reduces ventilation-perfusion inequalities, may be inhibited by inhalation anesthetics. In its absence, mismatch of ventilation and perfusion in both dependent and nondependent zones of the lungs will increase. (The magnitude of inhibition of hypoxic pulmonary vasoconstriction by inhalation anesthetics is being debated. Clinical studies in patients undergoing single-lung anesthesia have demonstrated only minimal inhibition.)

3. Blood flow to nondependent zones of the lungs is impeded by gravitational force. If pulmonary hypotension is a complication following induction of anesthesia, blood flow to nondependent regions will likely decrease, and consequently $\dot{V}/\dot{Q}$ ratio in these regions will be higher than normal.

Effect of Mechanical Ventilation

In the supine position, abdominal contents act as a column of fluid, and the pressure against the diaphragm is highest in dependent zones. Following induction of anesthesia, there is cephalad displacement of the end-tidal position of the diaphragm; this displacement is most pronounced in these dependent regions. While most of the diaphragmatic movement occurs in these dependent regions during spontaneous breathing, diaphragmatic movement takes place mainly in nondependent regions during muscle paralysis and mechanical ventilation (Fig. 10–1). Therefore the effect of mechanical ventilation is an increase in the $\dot{V}/\dot{Q}$ ratio of non-

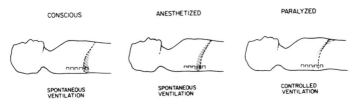

CONSCIOUS   ANESTHETIZED   PARALYZED

SPONTANEOUS   SPONTANEOUS   CONTROLLED
VENTILATION   VENTILATION   VENTILATION

FIGURE 10–1.   Excursion of the diaphragm, indicated by shaded areas, in conscious and anesthetized persons breathing spontaneously and in the paralyzed person ventilated mechanically. The dotted line marks the position of the diaphragm at the end of a normal expiration (i.e., at functional residual capacity) in a conscious person breathing spontaneously.

dependent zones at the expense of a fall in the $\dot{V}/\dot{Q}$ ratio of dependent zones. However the low $\dot{V}/\dot{Q}$ ratio of dependent zones during mechanical ventilation can be reversed by delivering a larger-than-normal tidal breath (50–100% above normal). During a large tidal exchange, a larger share of the tidal volume is delivered to dependent zones when alveoli in nondependent zones have reached the limit of their distensibility.

In addition, a longer inspiratory phase (i.e., a larger inspiration-expiration ratio) improves intrapulmonary distribution of gases and oxygenation. This is of special importance in patients with significant lung disease. However a prolonged inspiratory phase during positive-pressure ventilation can impede venous return, decrease cardiac output, and impair oxygenation (see "Oxygenation" below). In some critically ill patients, it may be necessary to monitor cardiac output while adjusting ventilatory parameters so as to obtain the best degree of oxygenation.

In summary, induction of anesthesia is accompanied by an increase in shunt-like effects as a result of falls in $\dot{V}/\dot{Q}$ ratio in dependent zones of the lungs. Similarly there is an increase in alveolar dead space as a result of increases in $\dot{V}/\dot{Q}$ ratio in nondependent zones.

AIRWAY RESISTANCE AND PULMONARY COMPLIANCE

Airway resistance (not including that due to anesthesia apparatus) can double during an uncomplicated anesthetic procedure. This increase is mainly due to reduction in the caliber of small airways following a fall in FRC. Similarly, pulmonary compliance has been observed to decrease during anesthesia. The significance of these changes is not clear.

CARBON DIOXIDE ELIMINATION

Arterial carbon dioxide tension ($PaCO_2$) in healthy conscious subjects lies between 36 and 40 mm Hg, but values approaching 70 mm Hg have been reported in anesthetized persons breathing spontaneously. This increase in $PaCO_2$ is a reflection of impairment of carbon dioxide elimination, even when the anesthetic is simple and uncomplicated.

Carbon dioxide elimination is directly proportional to alveolar ventilation. When alveolar ventilation falls, $PaCO_2$ rises. During anesthesia, not only is alveolar ventilation depressed (see "Alveolar Ventilation," above), but also "effective alveolar ventilation" is decreased (see "Ventilation-Perfusion Inequalities," above). In addition, ventilatory response to an increase in $PaCO_2$ is depressed by anesthetic agents (see "Control of Breathing," above). All of these factors contribute to carbon dioxide retention during anesthesia. Since carbon dioxide excretion can be increased by increasing ventilation, carbon dioxide retention can be rectified easily with larger tidal volumes delivered by either assisted or mechanical ventilation.

OXYGENATION

Oxygen tension of arterial blood (PaO_2) is 5–10 mm Hg below that of alveolar gas in healthy adults breathing room air. This alveolar-arterial oxygen tension difference is due to the presence of

1. An anatomic shunt, which is the venous return of bronchial and coronary circulations: It drains directly into the left heart and accounts for 2% of cardiac output.
2. Blood flow through areas of the lungs with a low $\dot{V}/\dot{Q}$ ratio: This accounts for approximately 3% of normal cardiac output.

It is well known that arterial oxygenation is impaired during anesthesia. This is reflected in the desaturation of arterial blood and in a larger-than-normal alveolar-arterial oxygen tension difference. The major cause of arterial desaturation during anesthesia is an increase in shunt-like effects of blood flowing through areas of the lungs with a low $\dot{V}/\dot{Q}$ ratio (see "Ventilation-Perfusion Inequalities," above).

Falls in cardiac output that are often seen during anesthesia also can contribute to impairment of arterial oxygenation. Figure 10–2 illustrates the mechanism of this impairment. A hypothetical patient "A" consumes oxygen at the rate of 200 ml/min and has a cardiac output of 5 L/min, of which 20%, or 1 L/min, is shunt. From each 100 ml of cardiac output 4 ml of oxygen must be

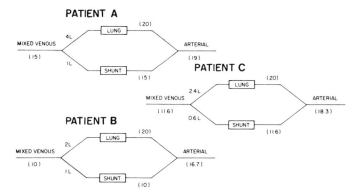

FIGURE 10–2. Effects of a fall in cardiac output on arterial oxygenation in hypothetical patients *A*, *B*, and *C*; see text for details. The oxygen content of blood (ml O_2/100 ml blood or volume percent) along each route is shown in parentheses.

extracted; the oxygen content of mixed venous blood is 15 ml O_2/100 ml blood. Blood going through the lungs is fully oxygenated and has an oxygen content of 20 ml/100 ml blood, but blood in the shunt has an oxygen content equal only to that of mixed venous blood. Therefore the arterial oxygen content is 19 ml O_2/100 ml blood.

In another patient, ''B,'' cardiac output has fallen to 3 L/min, but the shunt has remained fixed at 1 L/min. Since almost 6.7 ml of oxygen must be extracted from each 100 ml of cardiac output to satisfy the same oxygen consumption of 200 ml/min, mixed venous oxygen content has fallen to 10 ml O_2/100 ml blood. The outcome is a lower arterial oxygen content of 16.7 ml O_2/100 ml blood. Similar desaturation of arterial blood would have occurred even if the shunt fraction had remained at 20% of cardiac output. This is illustrated by patient ''C,'' whose cardiac output has fallen to 3 L/min but the shunt has fallen proportionately to 0.6 L/min. To satisfy oxygen demand, 6.7 ml of oxygen must be extracted from each 100 ml of arterial blood. As a result, mixed venous oxygen content has fallen to 11.6 ml O_2/100 ml blood, and arterial oxygen content, to 18.3 ml O_2/100 ml blood.

It is clear that desaturation of mixed venous blood is the underlying cause of impaired arterial oxygenation following a fall in cardiac output. This desaturation is also seen when the hemoglobin concentration is low or when there is a shift of the oxygen-hemoglobin dissociation curve to the left. These factors too may contribute to arterial hypoxemia in patients undergoing surgery.

Alveolar hypoventilation is another factor that can cause arterial desaturation in patients under anesthesia. This is because alveolar oxygen tension (P_AO_2) is determined not only by the oxygen tension of inspired gas (P_IO_2) but also by the carbon dioxide tension of alveolar gas (P_ACO_2). If the respiratory quotient is R, the relationship among these three variables can be expressed as

$$P_AO_2 = P_IO_2 - \frac{P_ACO_2}{R}$$

From this relationship it can be seen that an extremely high P_ACO_2 due to ventilatory depression can result in a low P_AO_2 and arterial hypoxemia.

PRACTICAL GUIDELINES

In addition to depression of ventilation, depression of ventilatory control, and increase in ventilation-perfusion inequalities following induction of anesthesia, cardiac output may fall under certain conditions. Although these changes are tolerated well by healthy young adults, they can cause serious hypercapnia and hypoxemia in ill patients. When hypercapnia is a complication of ventilatory depression, ventilation should be assisted or controlled. When hypoxemia is a complication of ventilation-perfusion mismatch, attention should be directed to improving the abnormal distribution of ventilation and perfusion. In general some or all of the following maneuvers can be tried:

1. Oxygenation of blood perfusing areas where the alveoli have a low $\dot{V}/\dot{Q}$ ratio can be improved by increasing the inspired oxygen fraction.

2. Ventilation to richly perfused dependent zones can be improved by minimizing forces that restrict the expansion of these regions (e.g., reducing the Trendelenburg tilt and removing unnecessary surgical packings).

3. During artificial respiration, ventilation of dependent zones can be improved with a larger-than-normal tidal breath. Mechanical dead space can be added to reduce the tendency of hypocapnia during large tidal-volume ventilation when necessary.

4. Application of positive end-expiratory pressure (PEEP) to increase functional residual capacity can improve the $\dot{V}/\dot{Q}$ ratio of dependent zones and improve arterial oxygenation. But PEEP can cause a fall in cardiac output by impeding venous return. Since a large drop in cardiac output can itself cause impairment of arterial oxygenation, the magnitude of PEEP should be appropriate in order to obtain a salutary effect.

5. During thoracotomy in the decubitus position, ventilation and

perfusion of the dependent lung can be improved by collapsing and packing the nondependent lung so that it is neither ventilated nor perfused.

Even if these measures fail, oxygen delivery can be improved by increasing cardiac output or the hemoglobin content of blood. When oxygen delivery to tissues is improved by either method, mixed venous blood will become less desaturated and arterial oxygenation will improve.

11

Anesthesia and Systemic Illness

The responsibility of the anesthesiologist would be simple indeed if all surgical patients were healthy. Unfortunately many have other illnesses that can complicate the course of anesthesia and subsequent recovery. Certain considerations are reason for concern:

1. Patients whose homeostatic mechanisms are ravaged by disease are very sensitive to the systemic side-effects of anesthesia.

2. Systemic illness can alter uptake, distribution, and elimination of anesthetic drugs.

3. Drugs used in the treatment of systemic illness can interact adversely with anesthetic agents.

4. Systemic illness can interfere with the execution of anesthetic procedures.

Therefore it is mandatory that all patients be carefully assessed and prepared before surgery. In general, no elective operations should be scheduled unless the patient is in the best possible state of health that is consistent with his organic illness. There is nearly always sufficient time for treatment to be instituted and take effect, even when an operation is urgent. In the following sections, risks associated with anesthesia in patients with some common illnesses are reviewed.

ISCHEMIC HEART DISEASE

Approximately 5% of the population in North America and western Europe has chronic myocardial ischemia. Affected patients are prone to have catastrophic cardiac complications during the operation and in the postoperative period, particularly if they have uncontrolled hypertension, congestive heart failure, major arrhythmias, respiratory failure, and hepatic or renal dysfunction.

These abnormalities should be brought under control before the scheduled operation. Patients with a history of myocardial infarction also deserve special attention, as they are at risk of having another infarction following surgery. According to the classic study reported by Tarhan and his colleagues in 1972, this risk is highest (36%) in patients whose previous infarction occurred 3 months or less before the operation; it is lower (16%) when the previous infarction occurred 4–6 months before the operation; and it is stable at 5% if the previous infarction occurred more than 6 months before the operation. Moreover the mortality rate is over 50% among patients who suffer recurrence of myocardial infarction in the perioperative period. Although a follow-up study reported in 1978 by the same group of authors showed essentially the same risks, Rao and associates showed in 1985 that outcome can be improved dramatically if invasive hemodynamic monitoring and aggressive treatment of hypertension and tachycardia (factors that can precipitate myocardial ischemia) are practiced. They reported a reinfarction rate of only 5.7% in patients who have a history of myocardial infarction within the last 3 months and a rate of 2.3% in those whose previous infarction occurred within the last 4–6 months. Therefore patients should not be exposed to the stress of anesthesia and surgery within 6 months of myocardial infarction if the operation is elective in nature. If the operation is urgent but not life threatening, a delay of 3 months is advisable. Only the life-threatening nature of a surgical illness justifies earlier operation. When early surgery is planned, aggressive measures to balance myocardial oxygen supply and demand are indicated.

If ischemic heart disease increases the anesthetic and surgical risk of these patients, drugs used in its treatment also give reason for concern. Cardiac glycosides used in the treatment of congestive heart failure or tachyarrhythmias are potentially toxic. During operation and in the postoperative period, many factors, including fluid and electrolyte shifts, acid-based abnormalities, hypoxemia, and abnormal renal and hepatic function, can precipitate life-threatening toxic complications. Therefore it is important to maintain normal oxygenation, normocapnia, and normal fluid, electrolyte, and acid-base balance in patients being treated with digitalis.

Diuretics used in the treatment of hypertension or fluid retention can cause hypokalemia by increasing urinary excretion of potassium. As a result, action of nondepolarizing muscle relaxants is prolonged, toxic side-effects of digitalis are increased, and the heart is more irritable. Serum potassium concentrations below 3 mEq/L should be corrected before the scheduled operation.

On the other hand, beta-adrenergic antagonists as well as calcium-channel blockers used in the treatment of arrhythmias, hypertension, or myocardial ischemia are myocardial depressants. Interaction between these agents and anesthetic drugs can cause bradycardia, hypotension, and congestive heart failure. But experience has shown that the myocardial depressant effects of these drugs and anesthetic agents are simply additive and predictable. Abrupt withdrawal of these drugs can precipitate an acute attack of coronary insufficiency and is contraindicated. Therefore maintenance therapy with beta-adrenergic antagonists or calcium-channel blockers should be continued right up to the time of surgery, unless there are signs of overdose.

The heart is an aerobic organ and relies entirely on oxidative metabolism to do work. During surgery in patients with ischemic heart disease, it is important to avoid complications that can increase myocardial work (e.g., tachycardia, hypertension, left ventricular failure, myocardial stimulation) or those that can decrease myocardial oxygen supply (e.g., hypotension, anemia, hypoxemia). Manipulation of circulatory dynamics and myocardial mechanics may be necessary to maintain a balance between myocardial oxygen demand and supply. In these situations, invasive monitoring is indicated (see "Invasive Hemodynamic Monitoring" in Chap. 14).

ESSENTIAL HYPERTENSION

Arterial hypertension is a manifestation of many organic disorders: renal failure, endocrine disorders (e.g., pheochromocytoma, Cushing's syndrome, primary aldosteronism), coarctation of the aorta, and toxemia of pregnancy; however, in approximately 80% of patients affected by hypertension no cause can be established. These patients are said to have primary essential hypertension. Many develop end-organ dysfunction (e.g., encephalopathy, nephropathy, heart failure) if the hypertension is not brought under control.

Many agents—diuretics, sympatholytic agents, calcium-channel blockers, direct-acting vasodilators; rauwolfia alkaloids—are used to treat hypertension. Management of affected patients has been influenced in the past by reports of severe hypotension and bradycardia during anesthesia. These complications were attributed to interactions between antihypertensive drugs and anesthetic agents. Therefore past practice was to stop all antihypertensive drugs for 1–2 weeks before the scheduled operation.

Current experience has shown that the danger of uncontrolled hypertension is worse than that of drug interaction. With careful titration of anesthetic drugs, circulatory complications are now rare in hypertensive patients even if their medications are continued right up to the time of operation. While these patients are being prepared for anesthesia and surgery, end-organ complications should be brought under control, hypokalemia caused by diuretics should be corrected, and the dose of sympatholytic agents, calcium-channel blockers, or vasodilators should be reviewed if disabling orthostatic hypotension or bradycardia (signs of an excessive dose) develops. If control of blood pressure is optimal, the treatment regimen should continue.

COMMON COLD

The common cold is a viral infection of the upper respiratory tract. Those who are afflicted have an irritable airway and so are more prone to develop bronchospasm and laryngospasm in response to instrumentation in the pharynx and larynx. Although no serious consequence has been observed following operations on the extremities, this is not true for abdominal procedures, even when they are minor (e.g., inguinal hernia repair). Guarding of the painful abdominal wound will decrease respiratory excursion, impair clearing of secretions, and increase the risk of respiratory complications; constant coughing in the early postoperative period, on the other hand, can disrupt the suture line. Common sense dictates that patients at the extremes of age and those who are afflicted with chronic illness should not be exposed to anesthesia and surgery when they are debilitated by viral infection. When incessant cough is accompanied by high fever, leukocytosis, and severe systemic manifestations, other infectious disease should be ruled out. In general a patient should recover completely from a cold before elective surgery is undertaken.

CHRONIC OBSTRUCTIVE LUNG DISEASE

Approximately 20% of adult males and 5% of adult females in North America and Western Europe have chronic generalized small airway disease, although most are not disabled. Cigarette smoking is without doubt a major cause of chronic airflow obstruction, and workers in polluted atmospheres (e.g., coal mines, farms, cotton mills) also have an obstructive component in their occupational lung disease. Afflicted patients have impaired pulmonary function that may be further compromised by ventilatory depression and deterioration of ventilation-perfusion inequalities under anesthesia. In the postoperative period, hypoventilation due to residual effects of anesthesia, guarding of painful surgical wounds, and recumbency can cause retention of secretion, atelectasis, and other pulmonary complications. These patients would benefit from careful preoperative evaluation and preparation.

Patients who are severely disabled should be admitted well in advance of the scheduled operation. All symptoms, signs, and progress of the disease should be documented, and a chest x-ray film should be ordered to exclude unsuspected active lesions. Other recommended laboratory investigations include arterial blood gas measurement and pulmonary function studies. While arterial blood gas measurement will yield useful information on overall respiratory function, pulmonary function tests can define the nature of abnormal function (restrictive versus obstructive) and delineate reversible components of abnormal function. Because it has no side-effects on respiratory function, regional anesthesia (if practical) is a real alternative to general anesthesia. The advantages and disadvantages of these techniques should be discussed with the patient.

To prepare these patients for surgery, regardless of whether regional or general anesthesia is planned, an active program aimed at improving respiratory function should be instituted. Breathing exercise, postural drainage, inhalation therapy with a mucolytic agent or bronchodilator, and incentive spirometry are helpful measures. All smokers have an irritable airway and a propensity to cough or develop bronchospasm and bronchorrhea following tracheal intubation or extubation. Refraining from smoking at this point is unlikely to eliminate this irritability, but it can reduce the amount of carboxyhemoglobin in the blood and improve oxygenation. (Carboxyhemoglobin concentration can be as high as 10% in heavy smokers.) Patients who are receiving bronchodilators should be allowed to continue their medication right up to the time of surgery, but the use of prophylactic antibiotics is not warranted.

LIVER DISEASE

The liver is a major depot from which drugs are eliminated. Intravenous anesthetics and narcotic analgesics are largely detoxified by hepatocytes; succinylcholine is broken down by plasma cholinesterase synthesized in the liver; and d-tubocurarine and pancuronium are partly secreted in the bile. Fortunately detoxification or excretion of these agents in most patients with liver disease is adequate unless hepatic damage is severe. A fall in serum albumin concentration and reversal of the albumin-globulin ratio are important indicators of altered drug sensitivity in liver disease. Requirements for drugs bound to albumin (e.g., thiopental) will be decreased, and requirements for drugs bound to globulin (e.g., d-tubocurarine) will be increased. Therefore it is important to titrate the dose of a drug against its effect in this group of patients. Furthermore attention should be directed to correction of biochemical and hematologic abnormalities and to avoidance of hepatotoxic agents.

Biochemical Abnormalities

Hyperbilirubinemia, hypoalbuminemia, and elevated levels of liver enzymes and ammonia are typical findings in patients with liver disease. Dilutional hyponatremia is frequently observed in patients with ascites and edema, although total body sodium may be above normal. Hypokalemia from excessive urinary loss is usually a sign of secondary aldosteronism. The glycogen store in the liver of patients suffering from fulminating hepatocellular damage is depleted; these patients can pass quickly into hypoglycemic coma. Yet many patients with chronic liver disease cannot cope with a carbohydrate load and have a glucose tolerance curve indistinguishable from that of diabetics. The need to maintain normoglycemia and fluid, electrolyte, and acid-base homeostasis in patients with liver disease is obvious.

Hematologic Abnormalities

Anemia due to hemolysis or chronic blood loss from esophageal varices is a common feature in patients with liver cirrhosis. Since these patients already have a hyperdynamic circulation, they tolerate blood loss poorly.

Coagulopathy is also a common complication of liver disease. Thrombocytopenia is the result of hypersplenism secondary to portal hypertension, and low titers of soluble factors II (prothrombin), V, VII, IX, and X, the result of decreased hepatic synthesis. Synthesis of factors II, VII, IX, and X is vitamin K dependent. These factors are deficient not only in hepatocellular disease but also in obstructive jaundice because absorption of fat-soluble vitamin K is impaired. Treatment of coagulopathy should be directed to replenishing these clotting factors. Platelet transfusion is indicated when platelet count falls below $50,000/mm^3$. Transfusion of fresh frozen plasma is indicated if prothrombin time is prolonged. Prolonged prothrombin time in patients with obstructive jaundice can be corrected with parenteral injection of vitamin K, but the salutary effect is not seen for 6–8 hours and can take 3 days.

Hepatotoxicity of Anesthetic Agents

There are clear indications that hepatic function is disturbed by both general and spinal anesthesia. Not only is hepatic blood flow depressed in the intraoperative period, but bromsulphalein (sodium sulfobromophthalein) clearance is decreased and liver enzyme levels are elevated in the postoperative period. However, intra-abdominal procedures can also cause reduction in liver blood flow, retention of bromsulphalein, and elevation of liver enzyme levels. Therefore the precise effect of anesthesia alone on liver function remains unclear. Halothane is the only agent that has clearly been identified as a potential hepatotoxin. Elevation of liver enzyme levels is increased both in frequency and in severity after repeated exposure to halothane, and cases of postoperative jaundice after halothane anesthesia have been reported. It is therefore only prudent to refrain from using halothane in patients with severe liver disease.

CHRONIC RENAL INSUFFICIENCY

Systemic complications are unavoidable in chronic renal insufficiency. With the advent of dialysis, uremic complications have become relics of the past. However, when patients with chronic renal failure require surgery, risks associated with hypertension, severe anemia, and fluid and electrolyte abnormalities cannot be ignored. Moreover, some anesthetics are nephrotoxic and others are eliminated only by the kidneys. Therefore choice of agents should be appropriate.

Hypertension

Not all patients with chronic renal failure are hypertensive, but when hypertension occurs it is mediated by overactivity of the angiotensin-renin system and exacerbated by hypervolemia. Elevated blood pressure may be difficult to control, and damage to end-organs (cardiomyopathy, encephalopathy, retinopathy) is a potential complication. Hemodynamic monitoring and aggressive treatment are indicated for these seriously ill patients.

Anemia in Chronic Renal Failure

Anemia of renal origin is resistant to conventional treatment, and repeated transfusion is neither practical nor advisable. Fortunately many affected patients have a normal cardiovascular and respiratory system and tolerate chronic anemia relatively well. Chronic anemia is not a contraindication to anesthesia and surgery unless there are other associated disabilities (see "Anemia" below).

Fluid and Electrolyte Abnormalities

Patients with abnormal renal function have difficulty excreting a fluid or electrolyte load. Although periodic dialysis can remove excess fluid and electrolytes, between dialyses these patients are vulnerable to the threat of hyperkalemia, hypernatremia, acidemia, and hypervolemia. Overzealous dialysis, on the other hand, can cause electrolyte and volume depletion. Therefore the records of dialysis should be reviewed so that abnormalities can be corrected.

In the presence of hyperkalemia, a further increase in serum potassium concentration following administration of succinylcholine can cause cardiac standstill (see "Increased Serum Potassium Concentration" in Chap. 5). If there is not enough time for dialysis, as in an emergency, sodium bicarbonate to correct acidemia, and cationic exchange resin, with or without glucose and insulin intravenously, to lower serum potassium concentration to normal values, should be given. Precurarization before the administration of succinylcholine also is helpful, but it does not eliminate altogether the possibility of a large rise in serum potassium concentration (see "Precurarization" in Chap. 5).

Nephrotoxicity of Anesthetic Agents

The kidney is another organ that is especially susceptible to the toxic effects of anesthetics and other drugs. Polyuric renal failure has been well documented in patients following methoxyflurane anesthesia. Nephrotoxicity is due to a high serum concentration of fluoride ions produced by metabolism of methoxyflurane. This agent is absolutely contraindicated in patients with chronic renal insufficiency. Enflurane, another fluorinated agent, has also been identified as potentially toxic to failing kidneys; however, this has been difficult to substantiate.

Renal Excretion of Muscle Relaxants

Like the liver, the kidneys play a major role in elimination of drugs. Since gallamine, metocurine, alcuronium, and decamethonium depend entirely on the kidneys for elimination, these agents' duration of action is related to the degree of the patient's renal impairment. They are absolutely contraindicated in functionally anephric patients, and they are relatively contraindicated in patients who have biochemical evidence of renal insufficiency.

DIABETES MELLITUS

Diabetes mellitus affects close to 2% of the general population. Not only can its systemic manifestations (generalized atherosclerosis, nephropathy, neuropathy, retinopathy) complicate anesthesia, but anesthesia and the consequence of surgery also can complicate the treatment of the underlying metabolic disorder. There are two diametrically opposing factors that can influence the control of carbohydrate metabolism in diabetic patients undergoing surgery. The natural response to the stress of surgery is an increase in blood sugar by glycogenolysis and gluconeogenesis, but at the same time the reduced caloric intake of surgical patients in the perioperative periods tends to lower blood sugar. Since anesthesia can mask the signs of hypoglycemia, it has been acceptable practice to allow diabetic patients to be slightly hyperglycemic but not ketotic during anesthesia and surgery.

Proper anesthetic and surgical management of diabetic patients depends on the treatment they receive. Patients with mature-onset diabetes that is treated by diet alone rarely require other than routine management. Those treated with oral hypoglycemic agents deserve more attention. In general, oral hypoglycemic agents should be discontinued on the day of the operation and for as long as caloric intake is reduced. (Note that the action of chlorpropamide can last well into the next day; patients on a reduced-caloric intake can become hypoglycemic up to 36 hours after receiving the last dose of this drug.) Fasting blood sugar concentration should be checked daily, and urine reaction should be checked every 4 hours during waking hours. Occasionally, administration of insulin in the perioperative period is necessary to obtain control, but this is uncommon.

Management of diabetics treated with insulin requires careful monitoring. Insulin-dependent diabetics are very sensitive to the reduction of caloric intake in the perioperative period and to the metabolic response to surgery. Ideally, elective operations for these patients should be scheduled in the morning. Like other patients scheduled for surgery, they should abstain from taking anything by mouth from midnight on the eve of the operation. On the morning of surgery, fasting blood sugar concentration should be checked, an intravenous infusion started, 5% dextrose in 0.45% saline infused at a rate of 100 ml/hour, and half the morning dose of insulin given subcutaneously. In the operating room, a 5% dextrose solution should be continued for maintenance, at a rate of 100 ml/hour, but third-space and other losses should be replaced with dextrose-free salt solutions (see also Chap. 20). During the operation and in the postoperative period, blood sugar concentration should be checked and regular insulin given according to this result or to urine reaction (the sliding-scale method). Depending on the surgical operation, daily insulin requirement may have to be adjusted even after caloric intake has returned to normal.

Hyperglycemia can cause impairment of leukocyte function and wound healing. Some anesthesiologists advocate tighter control of blood sugar level in insulin-dependent diabetics during the perioperative period; the aim is to maintain blood glucose level between 100 and 200 mg/100 ml. Many regimens have been proposed. A typical protocol follows:

1. Keep the patient n.p.o. from midnight.
2. Check fasting blood sugar concentration and start an intra-

venous infusion on the morning of the operation. Infuse 5% dextrose in 0.45% saline at the rate of 100 ml/hour.

3. Infuse regular insulin at a rate of 1 unit/hour simultaneously with the help of a constant infusion pump.

4. Repeat the measurement of blood sugar at 1- to 2-hour intervals and adjust the insulin infusion accordingly.

5. Replace other fluid loss with dextrose-free saline and add potassium chloride to the infusion as required.

ADRENOCORTICAL INSUFFICIENCY

Functional suppression of the adrenal cortex by chronic steroid therapy, rather than organic disease, is now the most common cause of adrenocortical insufficiency. The normal adrenal cortex secretes 20 mg of cortisol per day, and plasma level is approximately 14 μg/100 ml. Both this daily output and plasma level of cortisol increase in response to the stress of surgery, but they return to normal by the third postoperative day. It was long believed that the adrenal cortex required at least 2 years to recover its ability to respond to stress after discontinuation of chronic steroid therapy. Current experience indicates that the adrenal cortex can recover as early as a few weeks after withdrawal of chronic treatment. Steroid supplement is necessary only for patients who are currently on steroid therapy and for those whose therapy was discontinued within the last 2 months. In these patients, hydrocortisone hemisuccinate, 100 mg every 6 hours, should be started intramuscularly or intravenously on the day of operation and continued for 2 days postoperatively. If long-term therapy has been discontinued for more than 2 months, only careful observation is necessary. If signs of addisonian crisis become apparent, hydrocortisone should be given intravenously.

ANEMIA

Determination of hemoglobin concentration is an accepted routine in preoperative evaluation. A hemoglobin concentration below 10 g/100 ml is often considered a contraindication to anesthesia and surgery. However experience has shown that many anemic patients without cardiovascular, respiratory, and other systemic illnesses can tolerate anesthesia and surgery quite well. The reason for postponing an elective operation for an anemic patient is not simply the anemia but the fact that anemia is a common manifestation of other systemic maladies.

When anemia is discovered unexpectedly, its nature and cause should be fully investigated and treatment should be instituted before the operation. When the surgical illness is not causing the patient distress and the operation is truly elective, it is not unreasonable to postpone the operation until the patient responds to treatment. On the other hand, a hemoglobin concentration of less than 10 g/100 ml should not be regarded as an absolute contraindication to surgery. In fact, the surgical illness itself may be the cause of anemia, in which case the operation would be curative (e.g., vagotomy and pyloroplasty for duodenal ulcer; hysterectomy for metromenorrhagia).

It must be stressed that blood with a low hemoglobin concentration has a poor capacity for carrying oxygen, so cardiac output increases in anemic patients in order to maintain normal oxygen delivery. If it is necessary to proceed with surgery for such a patient, attention should be given to repletion of circulatory volume, maintenance of normal hemodynamics, and avoidance of arterial oxygen desaturation.

OBESITY

Severe obesity is a common nutritional problem among inhabitants of affluent countries. All obese patients have a smaller-than-normal FRC; a few also have hypoxemia and are prone to carbon dioxide retention (the pickwickian syndrome). Endocrine abnormalities (e.g., diabetes), hypertension, and heart failure are other associated complications.

Problems associated with anesthesia and surgery in the obese are related to size. Whereas the mildly to moderately obese patient requires minimal additional care, a morbidly obese patient challenges the wits of the operating room personnel. Even a simple procedure (e.g., transporting the patient to the operating room, positioning on the operating table, finding a mask or blood pressure cuff of the right size, or starting an intravenous infusion) can present an insurmountable problem. Intubation of the trachea can be difficult, and surgical access, nearly impossible. The obese patient is more likely to have gastric reflux while lying supine and is at increased risk for postoperative respiratory complications, deep vein thrombosis, and pulmonary embolism.

During evaluation, the morbidly obese patient should be checked routinely for pituitary, adrenal, thyroid, and islet cell dysfunction. Arterial blood gas and pulmonary function studies should be part of the preoperative laboratory investigation. A histamine H_2-receptor antagonist (e.g., cimetidine or ranitidine) should be prescribed to reduce the acidity and volume of gastric contents, and low-dose heparin to prevent deep vein thrombosis should be started on the day of operation and continued until the patient is fully ambulatory. During anesthesia and surgery, the airway should be protected with a cuffed endotracheal tube and ventilation should be controlled. Endotracheal intubation should be accomplished either with the patient awake or by rapid-sequence induction technique (see "Rapid-Sequence Induction" in Chap. 15). At the end of the operation, the endotracheal tube should be left in place until protective laryngeal reflexes have returned. In order to promote better ventilatory exchange, the patient should be nursed in Fowler's position if this is permissible. Deep breathing and coughing should be encouraged, and early ambulation is the best safeguard against deep vein thrombosis and pulmonary embolism.

ARTHRITIS

Approximately 3% of the general population are afflicted with arthritis, and more than one tenth of them are partially or totally disabled. While rheumatoid arthritis is more common among females and usually involves peripheral joints, ankylosing spondylitis is more common among males and involves axial joints. Both are systemic illnesses with other manifestations (e.g., anemia and pulmonary fibrosis in rheumatoid arthritis, aortic regurgitation and conduction abnormalities in ankylosing spondylitis).

Arthritis can be the cause of many difficulties in the operating room. Crippling skeletal deformities can make it difficult to position the patient on the operating table, and stiffness of the temporomandibular joints and the cervical spine can make direct laryngoscopy and tracheal intubation nearly impossible. Involvement of synovial joints of the larynx limits the choice of endotracheal tubes to smaller sizes, and fusion of costovertebral joints may be a cause of respiratory insufficiency under anesthesia. Therefore all the joints involved should be noted, and a plan should be devised to cope with these difficulties before induction of anesthesia. Obviously, systemic complications also should be investigated and abnormalities should be corrected before the operation. Since many arthritis patients are on long-term steroid treatment, it is important to review their steroid requirement in the perioperative period (see "Adrenocortical Insufficiency" above).

ALCOHOL AND DRUG ABUSE

Alcoholism is more than a social problem. Liver cirrhosis is a common complication in all alcoholics; beriberi heart disease due to thiamine deficiency is found in the malnourished; and alcoholic cardiomyopathy is an entity found in well-nourished alcoholics. Encephalopathy and poor vasomotor control caused by autonomic dysfunction (a consequence of peripheral neuropathy) are other important complications of chronic alcohol abuse. The patient who is acutely intoxicated tends to have a low gastric pH and a large volume of gastric contents. Since alcohol acts as a diuretic by inhibiting the secretion of antidiuretic hormone, dehydration may be also a problem. In addition significant hypoglycemia may be present during recovery from inebriation.

Anesthesia requirements vary among alcoholic patients. Since cross-tolerance exists between many central nervous system depressants, chronic alcoholics who are not acutely intoxicated require a larger-than-normal dose of both intravenous anesthetics for induction and of inhalation anesthetics for maintenance. On the other hand, the depressant effects of alcohol, anesthetics, and narcotic analgesics are additive. Therefore anesthesia requirements are lower than normal in acutely intoxicated persons. Alcoholics who have autonomic dysfunction are very sensitive to the circulatory depressant action of anesthetics, whether they are acutely intoxicated or not. A large drop in blood pressure without compensatory tachycardia during positive-pressure ventilation is another feature seen in these patients. If hypotension is severe, expansion of the intravascular volume is indicated, and treatment with an alpha-adrenergic agonist may be necessary (e.g., phenylephrine).

Besides abuse of alcohol, abuse of drugs is a growing problem in the more tolerant "new society"; a large number of illicit drugs are available. *Heroin addiction* in particular is a common problem in many large cities. Since all street drugs are of questionable purity, addicts may present with problems other than drug dependency: granulomatous lesions in the lungs, septicemia, subacute bacterial endocarditis of the triscupid and pulmonic valves. All intravenous drug addicts are at risk for hepatitis B infection and acquired immunodeficiency syndrome (AIDS); blood and body fluid precautions outlined in Chapter 25 should be practiced when anesthetizing these patients.

While it is not unreasonable to postpone elective operations until successful withdrawal is achieved, emergency operations cannot be delayed and no attempts at withdrawal should be made until recovery from surgery is complete. Heroin addiction is not a contraindication to general anesthesia or to regional techniques. However, opioids having both agonist and antagonist actions should not be used because they can precipitate the withdrawal syndrome. Methadone is the analgesic of choice. It is as potent as heroin and has a duration of action of up to 12 hours. The dose should be large enough to match the quantity of heroin habitually used.

In addition to their dependency, many addicts have adrenocortical insufficiency. Although prophylactic administration of steroids is not indicated, addisonian crisis may be the cause of unexplained hypotension during an otherwise uneventful anesthesia. Sudden withdrawal is another cause of unexplained hypotension in addicts. Hydrocortisone and methadone should be given intravenously when indicated.

The labile circulatory function of addicts underlines the importance of establishing an intravenous infusion before inducing anesthesia. Owing to absence of suitable superficial veins on the extremities, cannulation of a central vein may be the only recourse.

Cocaine, another street drug that is gaining popularity, is a stimulant. Sudden withdrawal causes paranoid ideation, delirium, insomnia, lassitude, and depression, but it is not life threatening. Cocaine addicts who snort, smoke, or inhale the drugs can present with unique airway problems from damage to mucosal linings of the respiratory tract and the lungs caused by intense vasocontriction. Like heroin addicts, those who inject cocaine intravenously are potential victims of hepatitis B infection, AIDS, and septicemia.

Acute cocaine intoxication is characterized by central nervous system irritability (restlessness, delirium, seizures) and increased sympathetic activity (tachycardia, hypertension, mydriasis). The intoxicated may present with tachyarrhythmias and myocardial ischemia, and some develop a hyperpyrexic, hypermetabolic state not unlike that seen in malignant hyperthermia. Since cocaine is broken down in plasma by cholinesterase, patients who have atypical plasma cholinesterase are particularly susceptible to this drug.

Many cocaine addicts are dependent on one or more central nervous system depressants as well in order to alleviate the undesirable side-effects of central nervous system stimulation. Such mixed addiction can present the clinician with a therapeutic challenge. It is important to recognize all of a patient's habits before prescribing treatment.

12

Preoperative Assessment and Preparation of the Patient

In anesthesia practice, "preparation" has two different meanings. In one sense, it means evaluation and care of the patient so that he or she is in the best possible state of good health before coming to the operating room; in the other, it means anticipation by the anesthesiologist of any possible complications during the operation or in the postoperative period. Adequate preparation in either sense cannot be achieved without knowledge of the patient's organic illness. Therefore a careful history should be obtained and the patient should be examined before the scheduled operation, as will be described in the following sections.

PREOPERATIVE ASSESSMENT

The Anesthetic History and Examination

Cases of mistaken identity and misdirected surgery are not just horror stories. They are true! Prevention of these mishaps begins with the preoperative visit. Each patient should be identified by name, date of birth, and hospital number. Information on the identification bracelet worn by the patient should be checked against that on the operating room schedule and the patient's chart. The patient should be questioned about the nature and site of the intended operation. Such confirmation can be obtained unobtrusively during the course of introduction. A tactful approach is the best way to establish rapport with the patient.

During the interview, the patient's medical history and progress in hospital should be reviewed. Special attention should be given to previous exposure to anesthesia, medication and treatment, allergies and atopy, personal habits, state of dentition, the airway, and concurrent illness.

At the conclusion of the interview, the patient should be allowed to ask questions. Many patients express concern or even fear of what is to come, indicating the need for psychological support. Words of reassurance are the best medicine to alleviate anxiety.

Previous Exposure to Anesthesia.   A history of previous exposure to anesthesia, with dates and agents used as well as known adverse reactions, should be recorded for the following reasons:

1. Exposure to halothane should not be repeated within 3 months.

2. Agents that have caused problems in the past should be avoided (e.g., succinylcholine causing prolonged apnea).

3. There may be a history of previous difficulties, such as difficult intubation or awareness during anesthesia.

Some patients may describe side-effects (e.g., nausea and vomiting or muscle pain) as complications, but obtaining a detailed history of the event will help to make clear the distinction. It is also worthwhile to note adverse reactions to anesthesia among family members because both atypical plasma cholinesterase and malignant hyperthermia are genetically determined (see "Atypical Plasma Cholinesterase" in Chap. 5 and "Malignant Hyperthermia" in Chap. 16).

Medication and Treatment.   It is essential to obtain complete information about past and present medication in the medical history. A knowledge of present medication is especially important in order to anticipate interaction with anesthetic agents. It has been the practice in the past to discontinue vasoactive and psychotropic agents before elective operations. Current experience has shown that patients are in a better position to cope if treatment they receive is optimal. These drugs are no longer discontinued before elective operations.

Allergies and Atopy.   All pharmaceutical agents are potential allergens. Obtaining a history of known allergies before prescribing a drug is a basic principle that should not be violated. Many patients may refer to a drug's side-effect as an allergic reaction (e.g., dyspepsia from salicylate compounds); these patients should be questioned carefully about the details of the event in order to differentiate a true allergic reaction from side-effect.

State of Dentition.   The upper incisors are vulnerable to damage by instrumentation during anesthesia (e.g., direct laryngoscopy). A note on the state of dentition—the presence of chips or cracks on the enamel, loose teeth, dentures, and crowns—can be important for future reference. The possibility of accidental damage to crowns made of procelain or synthetic material, no matter how remote this possibility may be, should be made clear; patients who are forewarned are more likely to accept the consequence without attributing blame.

The Airway.   Although tracheal intubation may not be planned for the anesthetic, the patient should nevertheless be examined for features that can make this procedure difficult because of possible need for emergency intubation in case of complications. Features of the head and neck that can make direct laryngoscopy and tracheal intubation difficult include prominent upper incisors, protruding or receding chin, stiffness of the temporomandibular joint or cervical spine, a short, thick neck, disease of the pharynx or larynx, and deviation of the trachea from midline. If nasotracheal intubation is contemplated, the patency of nasal passages should be confirmed also. In general, features that can give rise to difficulties in tracheal intubation can also render maintenance of a patent airway by mask difficult.

Concurrent Illness.   Many patients have other medical illnesses that can complicate the course of anesthesia and surgery. This subject has been reviewed in Chapter 11.

Laboratory Tests

Laboratory tests should be ordered only when indicated by the patient's medical history, physical findings, and intended surgery, to clarify the diagnosis and to follow progress after treatment. Many institutions also insist on certain standard laboratory tests on all surgical patients, even when they show no symptoms or signs of systemic illness (e.g., hemoglobin concentration or hematocrit and urinalysis on all patients, 12-lead electrocardiogram (ECG) on patients older than 40 years).

Fitness for Anesthesia

Is the patient "fit" for anesthesia? This is a question that must be asked at the end of the preanesthetic examination. But what is "fitness" for anesthesia?

It is known that the systemic side-effects of anesthesia can compromise vital functions. It is also known that abnormalities in systemic functions can affect the action and uptake, distribution, and elimination of anesthetic drugs. In short, healthy patients are less likely to have anesthetic complications. In this sense, "fitness" means good health. However there cannot be a single criterion of fitness; otherwise no surgical patient with concurrent medical illness would ever be able to reap the benefit of an operation. In general, a patient is an acceptable candidate for anesthesia and surgery if he is in the *best possible state of good health that is consistent with his organic illness*.

Although good health is the criterion of fitness, nature of the surgical procedure is the overriding factor in determining the timing of an operation. Elective surgery can be postponed indefinitely if time is required to improve the condition of an "unfit" patient. But if the operation will cure the "unfitness," or if it is urgent, then unnecessary delay should be avoided. For example, a child who is having respiratory difficulty is unfit. However, if distress is due to the presence of a foreign body in the bronchus, then its removal via a bronchoscope is curative; there is no reason for procrastination. Similarly a patient in congestive heart failure who requires urgent surgery to revascularize an ischemic leg is equally unfit. In this case, however, a little time well spent is necessary to bring heart failure under control. An aggressive approach to treatment can bring remarkable results, even in a short time.

Therefore fitness is only relative. It is a decision to be made jointly between the anesthesiologist and surgeon. Colleagues in other specialties may have to be consulted, but the anesthesiologist cannot forsake his part of the responsibility. In determining fitness, it is helpful to ask the following questions:

1. Does the patient have abnormal systemic function?
2. What is the underlying cause of the abnormality?
3. Can it be improved with treatment?
4. What is the treatment?
5. How much time is available for treatment to take effect?

If the answer to Question 3 is affirmative, then treatment should be initiated immediately to improve the patient's systemic function to an optimum within the time available.

Classification of Physical Status

All patients should be classified according to their physical capacity as part of the preoperative evaluation. The most common classification of physical status in use is that recommended by the American Society of Anesthesiologists:

Class I	A fit and healthy patient.
Class II	A patient with mild systemic illness.
Class III	A patient with severe systemic illness that is not incapacitating.
Class IV	A patient with an incapacitating systemic illness that is a constant threat to life.
Class V	A moribund patient who is not expected to live for more than 24 hours, with or without surgery.

In addition to this rating, the letter "E" should be entered if the operation is an emergency.

This classification of physical status is not a predictor of anesthetic risk because the insult of anesthesia cannot be divorced from that of surgery. However, attempts in arriving at a classification do serve at least two important purposes:

1. It ensures that the attending anesthesiologist has a clear overview of the patient's general state of health, without which an attempt at classification would be impossible.

2. It allows proper selection of patients for outpatient surgery. All Class I patients are suitable candidates, but only those in Class II or III whose systemic illness and its treatment are not complicated by the procedure are acceptable (see "The Ambulatory Patient" in Chap. 19).

PREPARATION OF THE PATIENT

Oral Intake Before Anesthesia

The protective laryngeal reflex is obtunded during anesthesia. Regurgitation of stomach contents and soiling of the airway are major risks in anesthetized patients. In order to minimize this risk, all patients scheduled for an elective operation should abstain from oral intake for at least 4–6 hours before induction of anesthesia. In general most adult patients are asked to abstain from taking anything by mouth from midnight before the day of operation except oral medication with a small amount of water.

Total reliance on a fixed time interval for gastric emptying can be misleading. Patients who have gastric stasis owing to disorders of the gastrointestinal tract and obstetric patients who are at term can have a large volume of gastric contents even after a prolonged fast. Similarly the stomach of traumatized patients empties slowly; food ingested before the accident can stay in the stomach for a long time. If incomplete gastric emptying is suspected, other means of protecting the airway should be planned (see "Rapid-Sequence Induction" in Chap. 15).

Premedications

The practice of premedication (preanesthetic medication) is rooted in the era of ether anesthesia. The traditional indications were alleviation of anxiety, facilitation of the induction of anesthesia, reduction of salivary and bronchial secretions, and minimizing anesthetic requirement. Drugs commonly used were sedatives (e.g., barbiturates), antisialagogues (e.g., atropine or hyoscine), and narcotic analgesics (e.g., morphine, meperidine, or pantopon).

With modern anesthetic techniques, however, induction of anesthesia is smooth and pleasant; copious salivary and bronchial secretions are rare; anesthetic requirement can be adjusted as the needs arise. Times have changed and so has the reason for premedication. It is still indicated for the relief of anxiety, but some new indications have emerged, including protection against acid aspiration penumonitis and prophylaxis against other complications.

Relief of Anxiety. Anxiety is a natural reaction when one is faced with uncertainty. There is no better anxiolytic agent than words of understanding, support, and reassurance. This puts emphasis on the importance of establishing rapport with and gaining the confidence of the patient during the preoperative visit. For the patient who needs it, the prescription of a tranquilizer (e.g., 10–15 mg of diazepam orally or 2–4 mg of lorazepam sublingually, given 1–2 hours before the scheduled operation) is more appropriate than a sedative. If anxiety is due to pain, a potent analgesic should be prescribed also.

Protection Against Acid Aspiration Pneumonitis. Aspiration of gastric contents during anesthesia is a major cause of morbidity. As little as 25 ml of gastric juice with a pH of 2.5 or less is enough to produce acid pneumonitis. Some patients' basal gastric contents may well exceed these limits despite overnight fasting; if so, they are at risk of regurgitation and aspiration. Therefore many methods of modifying this volume and acidity with pharmacologic agents have been proposed, including:

1. Neutralizing gastric juice with antacid before induction of anesthesia (e.g., 30 ml of $\frac{1}{3}$ molar sodium bicitrate).

2. Giving histamine H_2-receptor antagonist (e.g., 300 mg cimetidine or 150 mg ranitidine) orally the night before and 1–2 hours before induction of anesthesia, to reduce both the acidity and volume of gastric contents.

3. Giving 20 mg metoclopramide orally $\frac{1}{2}$–2 hours before induction of anesthesia, to encourage gastric emptying.

It must be stressed that these methods of modifying gastric volume and acidity are only added safety measures. They are not meant to supplant rapid-sequence induction in susceptible patients (see "Rapid-Sequence Induction" in Chap. 15).

Prophylaxis Against Other Complications. Some anesthetic side-effects or complications can be prevented by other drugs given before induction of anesthesia. These drugs should be included as premedication, if indicated. They include antiemetics (e.g, prochlorperazine) for patients prone to nausea and vomiting, antihistamines (e.g., chlorpheniramine) for atopic persons, hydrocortisone for patients on chronic steroid therapy, and dantrolene for suspected victims of malignant hyperthermia. In addition, patients who are receiving antianginal, antihypertensive, and antiarrhythmic drugs or bronchodilators should be allowed to continue with their medication right up to the time of surgery.

13

Direct Laryngoscopy and Tracheal Intubation

Tracheal intubation was first described in humans in 1788, when it was recommended for resuscitation of drowning victims, but another century elapsed before the procedure was introduced into anesthesia practice. Tracheal intubation is a safe procedure that allows direct access to the airway; in skilled hands it has few serious complications. These advantages have contributed to the popularity of endotracheal anesthesia. However, endotracheal tubes can become kinked, compressed, or dislodged. The presence of an endotracheal tube does not guarantee a clear airway. Continuous vigilance is still required.

INDICATIONS

Indications for tracheal intubation in anesthesia practice are as follows:

1. *Maintenance of a patent airway*
   a. When an awkward intraoperative position is required (e.g., lateral decubitus, prone, sitting)
   b. When the airway is inaccessible (e.g., during head and neck operations)
   c. When difficulties with the face mask are anticipated (e.g., in grossly obese or edentulous patients or those with unusual facial features)
2. *Protection of the airway* from contamination by blood, pus, debris, or stomach contents
3. Use of *controlled ventilation* as part of the anesthetic technique. (Controlled ventilation is safe only if an endotracheal tube is in place. While it is permissible to ventilate the lungs via a face mask for short periods, as before tracheal intubation, continuation over a longer period can lead to gastric distension and regurgitation.)

In addition, tracheal intubation is practiced outside the operating room for tracheobronchial toilet, to protect the airway of an unconscious patient, for patients who require ventilatory assistance, and during cardiopulmonary resuscitation. All medical practitioners should be thoroughly familiar with the technique.

EQUIPMENT

Pharyngeal Airways

The tongue of an unconscious patient who is lying supine tends to fall backward and to occlude the glottic opening. Pharyngeal airways are molded tubes inserted through the nose or mouth to keep the airway patent (Fig. 13–1A, B). Nasopharyngeal airways made of latex rubber are soft and supple. Oropharyngeal airways, which are made of plastic, are more rigid and can also be used to prevent semiconscious patients from biting on the endotracheal tube, thus occluding its lumen. Both come in various sizes.

Modified oropharyngeal airways are availble also for fiberoptic laryngoscopy and intubation via the orotracheal route (Fig. 13–1C, D). The Williams intubating airway has a large-bore lumen that can accommodate an endotracheal tube, and the Berman airway has a slit along its entire length. The functions of these special airways are explained in "Fiberoptic Laryngoscopy and Intubation" below.

Laryngoscopes

The laryngoscope is an instrument used for direct inspection of the larynx. Conventional laryngoscopes used by anesthesiologists have two separate components: a handle that provides housing for the batteries and a detachable and interchangeable blade with a light for illumination. There are two basic designs of laryngoscope blades (Fig. 13–2): curved (e.g., MacIntosh) and straight (e.g., Magill or Miller). All blades are available in different lengths suitable for use in neonates, children, or adults.

A fiberoptic laryngoscope made of flexible optical fibers is available for use when intubation is expected to be difficult (Fig. 13–3). By manipulating a lever on its handles, the operator can point its tip in all directions so as to obtain a view of the glottic opening otherwise not accessible through a rigid laryngoscope.

Endotracheal Tubes

Endotracheal tubes are made of either rubber or plastic (Fig. 13–4). Some are plain and shaped into a curve; some have metallic

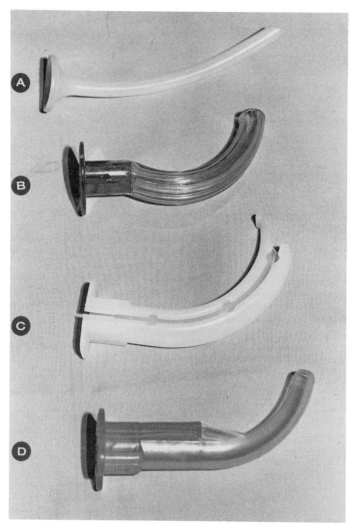

FIGURE 13–1.   Pharyngeal airways: nasopharyngeal airway, *A*, oropharyngeal airway, *B*, Berman intubating airway, *C*, and Williams intubating airway, *D*.

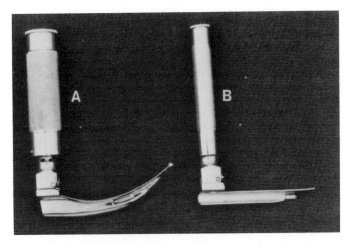

FIGURE 13–2. Laryngoscopes. *A*, A laryngoscope with the MacIntosh blade. *B*, A laryngoscope with a Magill-type blade.

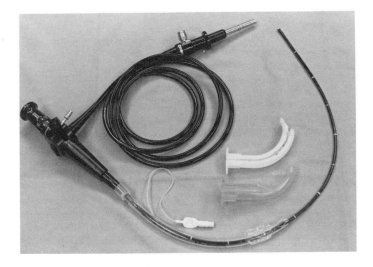

FIGURE 13–3. A fiberoptic bronchoscope shown with two intubating airways.

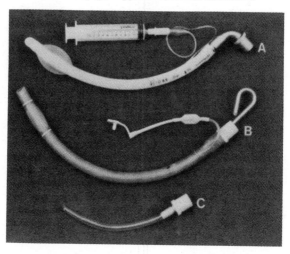

FIGURE 13–4. Endotracheal tubes. *A*, A plastic disposable endotracheal tube with a curved connector. *B*, A reinforced tube with a malleable stylet in its lumen. *C*, Cole's tube with a straight connector.

or nylon coils embedded in their wall to prevent kinking or compression; and some have a slim tracheal portion and a fat laryngeal portion so that the "shoulder" at the junction will limit advancement of the tube beyond the larynx and prevent inadvertent bronchial intubation. All tubes should be made of nontoxic and nonirritant material, and they should conform to certain basic designs. Endotracheal tubes that meet these standards bear the codes "IT" and "Z-79."

Most endotracheal tubes have an inflatable cuff near the distal end. Tubes without a cuff are used primarily in pediatric patients (see "The Pediatric Patient" in Chap. 19). The purpose of the cuff is to provide an air-tight seal between the outer wall of the tube and the trachea. By using a syringe, this cuff can be inflated with air via a separate catheter. A pilot balloon is incorporated into this catheter to indicate whether the cuff is inflated or deflated.

Several scales have been used in the past to indicate the physical dimensions of endotracheal tubes (the French, the Davol, and the Magill systems). In current practice the indicated size is the actual inner diameter in millimeters. In general, adult males require an 8- to 9-mm tube, and adult females, a 7- to 8-mm tube for orotracheal intubation. For nasotracheal intubation, the size of tubes should be reduced by 1–2 mm. In children, appropriate tube size can be estimated according to the formula

$$\frac{\text{Age in years}}{4} + 4.5 \text{ mm}$$

(The French scale, a system used to denote the outer dimension of tubular instruments, is still popular in parts of continental Europe. When the thickness of its wall is taken into account, the inner diameter of an endotracheal tube is roughly equivalent to its size in French units divided by 4.)

Selecting an endotracheal tube of correct length is as important as selecting one of correct size. There are many ways to estimate the correct length of an endotracheal tube. A popular one based on anatomic landmarks is to measure the distance between the ear lobe and the corner of the mouth on the same side of the face. An orotracheal tube should be cut to twice this length, and a nasotracheal tube, to 2 cm longer. The correct length of the selected tube can be confirmed by placing it alongside the patient's face and neck. An endotracheal tube of the correct length should extend from the lower incisor or the nose to a point midway between the cricoid cartilage and Louis's angle (the sternal angle).

Intubating Forceps

During nasotracheal intubation, it is difficult to manipulate the tip of the endotracheal tube. Magill forceps (Fig. 13–5A) are designed specifically for the purpose of guiding the end of the en-

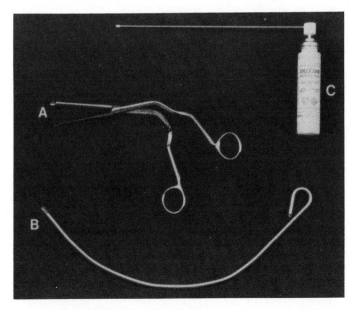

FIGURE 13–5.   Endotracheal equipment. *A*, Magill intubating forceps. *B*, The malleable stylet. *C*, The laryngeal spray.

dotracheal tube through the glottic opening. They are also helpful in placing nasogastric tubes under direct vision.

Malleable Stylet

The stylet is a thin piece of metal or plastic than can be threaded through the lumen of an endotracheal tube (Fig. 13–5B). It is a useful aid when exposure of the larynx is difficult. Being malleable, it can be used to shape the endotracheal tube into curves that will facilitate intubation. A stylet should be lubricated well so that it can be introduced and withdrawn with ease.

Laryngeal Spray

The laryngeal spray is designed to nebulize a fixed dose of local anesthetic solution (usually lidocaine) and deposit it on the mucosal surface of the larynx and trachea (Fig. 13–5C). This method of topical anesthesia is necessary if intubation of a conscious patient is attempted. It is said that topical anesthesia can attenuate reflexes provoked by tracheal intubation (e.g., arrhythmias, hypertension, laryngospasm). Although the issue is controversial, some anesthesiologists routinely spray the cords and trachea with a local anesthetic solution before tracheal intubation, even after general anesthesia has been induced.

Lubricant

Lubrication of orotracheal tubes is optional, but nasotracheal tubes and stylets should always be lubricated with water-soluble jelly or ointment, with or without lidocaine. Products containing oil can cause lipid pneumonia. (Some anesthesiologists believe that use of a local anesthetic lubricant can minimize tissue irritation and the incidence of sore throat.)

TECHNIQUES OF INTUBATION

Planning and preparation are vital in all aspects of anesthesia, and tracheal intubation is no exception. During the preoperative visit, the patient should be examined for features that can make tracheal intubation difficult (see "The Airway" in Chap. 12). Before an attempt at intubation is made, the following preparations are mandatory:

1. Verify that the anesthetic machine and its accessories are in working order (see Chap. 15).
2. Select an endotracheal tube of appropriate size and cut it to the appropriate length. Confirm the integrity of its cuff and make

sure that it has the right connector for the anesthetic circuit. (Since size cannot be accurately judged, endotracheal tubes 0.5 mm larger and smaller than the estimated size should also be readily available.)

3. Ascertain that the laryngoscope is in working order.

4. Check that the cuff inflator, intubating forceps, malleable stylet, and laryngeal spray are readily available and easily accessible.

5. Ascertain that the means of pharyngeal suction is available on demand.

6. Have a trained person available to give assistance.

Posture of the Head and Neck

The correct posture of the head and neck for direct laryngoscopy is the same, regardless of the type of laryngoscope blade used or the route of intubation; the position is characterized by flexion of the cervical spine and extension of the head at the atlanto-occipital joint (tip the head backward while it is resting comfortably on a pillow). When the head and neck are correctly positioned, the long axes of the oral cavity, pharynx, and trachea lie almost in a straight line (Fig. 13–6A). Incorrect positioning of the head and neck is the most common cause of difficult intubation. A mistake made by many beginners is to extend the head and neck fully.

Orotracheal Intubation

Endotracheal intubation, whether by the orotracheal or the nasotracheal route, is a skill that can be acquired only through practice. However, a few words of advice for beginners are helpful. The following steps describe the technique of orotracheal intubation using a curved blade:

1. Position the patient's head correctly on a pillow.

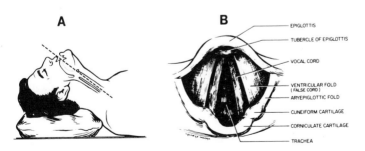

FIGURE 13–6. Technique of tracheal intubation. A, Correct posture of the head and neck. B, A view of the glottis through the laryngoscope.

2. Hold the laryngoscope in the palm of the left hand and introduce the blade into the right side of the patient's mouth. Advance the blade posteriorly and toward the midline, sweeping the tongue to the left and holding it away from the visual path with the flange of the blade while doing so. *Check that the lower lip is not caught between the lower incisors and the laryngoscope blade.*

3. When the epiglottis is in view, advance the tip of the laryngoscope blade into the vallecula formed by the base of the tongue and the epiglottis. *Check that the upper lip is not caught between the upper incisors and the laryngoscope blade.*

4. Lift the laryngoscope upward and forward, in the direction of the long axis of the handle, to bring the larynx into view. If the epiglottis is seen to overhang the larynx, advance the tip of the blade further into the vallecula. If the esophagus is in sight, withdraw the blade until the larynx falls into view. (A common mistake made by inexperienced operators at this point is to use the upper incisors as a fulcrum for leverage. This not only damages the upper incisors but also pushes the larynx out of sight.)

5. When the larynx is in view (Fig. 13–6*B*), introduce the endotracheal tube from the right with its concave curve facing downward (caudad) and the right side of the patient. Have the assistant retract the angle of the patient's mouth on the right side if room is required to maneuver the endotracheal tube into the larynx. (Another common mistake made by the beginner is to obstruct his own view by introducing the endotracheal tube centrally, along the curve of the laryngoscope blade.)

6. If only the posterior aspect of the glottis (the arytenoids) is in view, have the assistant apply gentle backward pressure on the thyroid cartilage so that the larynx can be brought into full view. (An alternative is to use the stylet or the intubating forceps to direct the tip of the endotracheal tube into the anterior larynx.)

7. Once the endotracheal tube is in place, apply positive-pressure ventilation to the lungs while the assistant inflates the cuff gradually until an airtight seal is obtained.

8. Continue to ventilate the lungs and rule out esophageal intubation by auscultation over both the chest wall and the epigastrium. (Auscultation over the chest wall alone should not be relied upon to verify the position of the endotracheal tube because noise of air moving down the esophagus may not be distinguishable from breath sounds. Air entering the stomach gives off a gurgling sound over the epigastrium that is unique. The most reliable method to confirm endotracheal intubation is capnography. Appearance of the expiratory carbon dioxide wave form rules out esophageal intubation.)

9. Rule out bronchial intubation by checking movement over the apices of the lungs and by auscultation over the apical and axillary regions of the chest wall. Unequal movement and unequal air entry are signs of bronchial intubation.

10. Fasten the endotracheal tube securely after its correct position is confirmed.

The technique of direct laryngoscopy and intubation using a straight laryngoscope blade is essentially similar. The only difference is that the blade should be slipped beneath the epiglottis so that it too is lifted upward and forward. Once the technique of direct laryngoscopy and intubation is mastered, the choice of blades becomes a matter of personal preference. In general, techniques that use curved blades are easier to learn and therefore more popular.

Nasotracheal Intubation

Orotracheal intubation is generally the method of choice in the operating room, but nasotracheal intubation is indicated for operations in the oral cavity. Use of the nasotracheal route for intubation requires some modifications to the technique described before:

1. Topical cocaine, 10%, or phenylephrine, 0.25%, should be applied to the nasal passages to shrink the muscosal lining before nasotracheal intubation is attempted.

2. The nasotracheal tube should be 2 cm longer and 1–2 mm smaller than the orotracheal tube.

3. A curved connector is more convenient than a straight connector.

4. The tube must be lubricated well.

5. The tube should be advanced through the nose directly backward (not cephalad) toward the nasopharynx. When it has been maneuvered into the pharynx, direct laryngoscopy is performed, as described, and the nasotracheal tube is guided into the glottis with a pair of intubating forceps.

6. Once the endotracheal tube is in place, the cuff is inflated, and esophageal and bronchial intubation ruled out, as described above.

Intubation Under Topical Anesthesia

Tracheal intubation for surgical procedures is usually done following induction of anesthesia and administration of a muscle relaxant. In a small number of cases intubation without the benefit of general anesthesia is indicated—specifically in patients in whom induction of anesthesia is considered unsafe unless the airway is secured first:

1. Patients with disease (tumors, trismus, trauma) affecting the patency of the airway

2. Patients in whom difficult intubation is anticipated

3. Patients with an unstable cervical spine (Manipulation of the head and neck in such patients can injure the spinal cord; response to pain in the awake state can warn the anesthesiologist of this trespass.)

"Awake intubation" can be attempted with the help of either conventional laryngoscopes or a fiberoptic scope. In either case the airway can be anesthetized with lidocaine according to these steps:

1. Use 10 ml of 2% viscous lidocaine as a mouthwash and gargle to anesthetize the oral cavity.

2. With the aid of the laryngoscope and a laryngeal spray, apply 100–150 mg of lidocaine to the larynx and trachea. Pay special attention to the piriform fossae, the vocal cords, and the trachea beyond the cords. (Two alternatives for anesthetizing the trachea topically are also effective. One method is to inject 5 ml of 2% lidocaine into the trachea through the cricothyroid membrane as follows: Raise a skin wheal and puncture the cricothyroid membrane with a 20-gauge intravenous cannula. Confirm that the tip of the needle is in the tracheal lumen by aspiration for air. Thread the plastic cannula into the tracheal lumen and withdraw the needle. Inject the solution quickly through the cannula during inspiration. Because of the risk of causing laceration to the trachea when the patient coughs in response to the injected lidocaine solution, use of a plain steel needle for this procedure is not recommended. Another method is to allow the patient to inhale 3–5 ml of nebulized 4% lidocaine. This procedure is time consuming; 20–30 minutes of inhalation via a properly fitted mask is required for best results.)

3. Anesthetize the nasal passage with topical cocaine if the nasal route is used.

"Awake intubation" is unpleasant for the patient. Time must be allowed for the topical anesthetic to take effect. Direct laryngoscopy should be done with skill and gentleness. Fentanyl, with or without diazepam, given intravenously for sedation, can be most helpful in securing the cooperation of the patient.

Fiberoptic Laryngoscopy and Intubation

This technique is particularly useful in difficult intubations or when manipulation of the head and neck is contraindicated (e.g., in fracture of the cervical spine). All practitioners of anesthesiology should acquire this skill; use of this technique by the inexperienced in an emergency is seldom successful.

When difficulty in visualizing the glottis with a conventional rigid laryngoscope is anticipated, fiberoptic laryngoscopy should be the method of choice rather than of last resort. Accumulation of secretions and blood from unsuccessful attempts at rigid laryngoscopy and intubation can make visualization of the larynx with the fiberoptic scope nearly impossible.

Both the nasal and the oral route can be used for this technique. In either case the airway should be anesthetized topically by one of the methods described earlier. The lubricated endotracheal tube should be threaded onto the lubricated stem of the scope, as illustrated in Figure 13–3, before the procedure. Suction applied to the suction port of the laryngoscope is also essential. When the nasotracheal route is used, the steps are:

1. Have the patient lying supine or sitting comfortably in semi-Fowler's position. (If the patient is sitting up, the operator should position himself at the subject's side, facing him. If the patient is lying supine, the operator can be positioned either at the subject's head or at his side.)

2. Advance the stem of the scope backward toward the nasopharynx through the nose until its tip has been positioned in the oropharynx.

3. Look through the scope and manipulate the tip of the stem as it is advanced in search of the epiglottis.

4. Ask an assistant to support the jaw and maneuver the tip of the scope to go past the epiglottis posteriorly in search of the glottis.

5. Advance the tip of the scope through the cords into the trachea. (Appearance of tracheal rings at this point will confirm that the tip of the scope is in the trachea. If the glottis has disappeared from view without the appearance of tracheal rings, the tip of the scope has advanced into the esophagus or lodged in the vallecula or piriform fossa. It should be withdrawn slowly until the epiglottis is again in view, when steps 4 and 5 are repeated.)

6. Once the tip of the scope is in place, advance the endotracheal tube into the trachea using the stem of the scope as guide.

7. Inflate the cuff of the endotracheal tube and verify its position, as described above.

The method of intubation via the orotracheal route is essentially similar, but either the Williams or Berman intubating airway should be used as a conduit for the laryngoscope and to prevent the patient from biting on the fragile stem of the scope. When the Tudor Williams airway is used, an endotracheal tube that is large enough to accommodate the stem of the scope but small enough to slip through the lumen of the airway should be selected. When the Berman airway is used, the stem of the scope should be slid out of the airway through its opening on the side once the trachea is entered.

EXTUBATION

Extubation is usually a simple, uncomplicated procedure when done properly. As with intubation, a certain routine should be followed (see also "Emergence" in Chap. 15):

1. Check that the patient has regained normal neuromuscular function if muscle relaxant was used (see "Monitoring Neuromuscular Function" in Chap. 14) and check that the patient is recovering from the effects of anesthesia and is breathing spontaneously with adequate volumes.

2. Allow the patient to breathe 100% oxygen at high flow for 2–3 minutes to wash out nitrous oxide.

3. Remove secretions accumulated in the pharynx by suction. If secretions are suspected in the tracheobronchial tree, remove them with a suction catheter introduced through the lumen of the endotracheal tube.

4. Check that the patient is not in a semiconscious state. Extubation at this plane can provoke laryngospasm.

5. Turn the patient onto his side if he is still unconscious.

6. Deflate the cuff and remove the endotracheal tube quickly but smoothly during inspiration.

7. Continue to give the patient oxygen as required.

COMPLICATIONS OF LARYNGOSCOPY AND INTUBATION

Complications following short-term tracheal intubation in the operating room are usually minor. The following problems may be encountered:

Trauma to Lips, Teeth, and Soft Tissues of the Airway. Constant awareness of the possibility of these complications and meticulous technique will help to reduce their incidence.

Reflex Tachycardia and Hypertension, Ventricular Arrhythmias, Bronchospasm, and Chest Wall Spasm. These complications are common when the trachea is intubated with the patient at a light plane of general anesthesia. The pressor response is attenuated by increasing the depth of anesthesia or by applying topical lidocaine to the larynx and trachea. The administration of lidocaine, 1.5 mg/kg intravenously, 1.5–3 minutes before the procedure is another alternative. Bronchospasm and chest wall spasm are also associated with intubating the trachea under light anesthesia. Bronchospasm usually responds to intravenous aminophylline, and chest wall spasm, to muscle relaxants.

Bronchial Intubation. Inadvertent bronchial intubation (usually of the right main bronchus) is a not an infrequent complication of tracheal intubation because methods of estimating the correct length of an endotracheal tube are only guides. Auscultation of the chest bilaterally for air entry is the only sure method for determining that the tube has been successfully placed in the trachea and not in a mainstem bronchus.

Laryngospasm Following Extubation. This problem is common when extubation is done with the patient in a semiconscious state. Extubation in adults should be done either in a relatively deep plane of anesthesia or when the protective laryngeal reflex has returned; extubation in children and infants should be done when laryngeal reflex has returned.

Post-intubation Hoarseness and Sore Throat. These unpleasant side-effects are due to the mechanical presence of the endotracheal tube. Use of low-pressure cuffs has not eliminated these problems entirely. In order to minimize them, unnecessary movement of the head and neck should be avoided once the endotracheal tube is in place.

Post-intubation Stridor or Croup. Pediatric patients are more prone to this complication than adults; it is due to edema of subglottic regions of the airway. These patients should be given humidified oxygen, and administration of racemic epinephrine by inhalation may be necessary. Selection of an endotracheal tube of the correct size will reduce the incidence of this complication (see also "Pediatric Patients" in Chap. 19).

Monitoring Principles and Practice

The primary goal of surgical anesthesia is to alleviate pain and stress. Unfortunately the patient is also exposed to the systemic side-effects of anesthetic drugs in the process and is rendered helpless against physiologic trespasses accompanying surgery. His survival is totally dependent on the supportive care provided by the anesthesiologist. Therefore, careful monitoring of the patient's vital functions and of the effects of anesthesia and surgery is mandatory.

To exercise the clinical skills of inspection, palpation, percussion, and auscultation is the most basic means of monitoring. In an attempt to improve on human senses, industry has made available a large array of automated instruments to measure body functions, to monitor the anesthesiologist's action and the patient's response, to detect failure in the anesthetic machine and its circuit, and to sound an alarm when certain limits have been exceeded. What is an appropriate level of monitoring during anesthesia? To answer this question requires a knowledge of the methods available and an understanding of their capabilities and limitations.

MONITORING DEPTH OF ANESTHESIA

Clinical Signs

Although they vary according to the agents used, clinical signs associated with surgical anesthesia remain a reliable gauge of the depth of anesthesia. When barbiturates are used for induction of anesthesia, loss of eyelash reflex (blinking in response to gentle stroking of the eyelash) marks the onset of unconsciousness. Some patients may yawn or take a deep breath just before falling into a deep sleep. When ketamine is used, unconsciousness is marked by the onset of a cataleptic state accompanied by profound analgesia. When volatile agents are used, the signs of surgical anesthesia include a central gaze, pupils that are small and reactive to light, and respiration that is regular in both rate and depth (automatic breathing).

The most critical test of depth of anesthesia is the patient's reaction to surgical stimulation. Somatic responses may take the form of frank movements of extremities or laryngospasm, or it may be subtle, as in wrinkling of the forehead, vocalization, irregular breathing, or breath holding. Sympathetic responses to surgical stimulation include hypertension, tachycardia, sweating, and lacrimation. Both somatic and sympathetic responses to surgical stimulation should be abolished by anesthesia in the patient who is breathing spontaneously. In the paralyzed patient, however, only sympathetic responses are available to help in gauging depth of anesthesia. In short, the patient who is adequately anesthetized is quiet, normotensive, warm, pink, and dry. A progressive fall in blood pressure and profound respiratory depression are signs of an excessive depth of anesthesia. Fixed dilated pupils are an ominous sign; immediate investigation is called for, and gross overdose or profound hypoxia must be ruled out.

Electroencephalogram

Two types of rhythms can be identified on classical 16-channel electroencephalogram (EEG) in normal adults: sinusoidal alpha waves of 8–12 Hz present over the occipital and parietal regions in relaxed subjects whose eyes are closed but disappear when eyes are opened; lower voltage beta waves of 13–30 Hz present over central and frontal regions. Slower theta rhythm (4–7 Hz), delta waves (less than 4 Hz), and electrical silence—present either focally or diffusely—are always abnormal in awake subjects and can be traced to destructive lesions. Certain general but nonspecific trends can be observed on EEG following induction of surgical anesthesia. They include the spread of alpha waves anteriorly over all parts of the cerebral cortex and appearance of theta and delta rhythm. Alpha waves predominate during deep levels of anesthesia, and electrical silence follows onset of barbiturate coma.

In order to facilitate the use of EEG monitoring by less experienced personnel in the operating suite, various electronic data processing techniques have been introduced to remove artifacts, analyze frequencies, quantify amplitudes, and report trends (e.g., by power spectral analysis). Use of computer-processed EEG to monitor depth of total intravenous anesthesia has been explored. However EEG changes associated with anesthesia do not reflect the tissue level of anesthetic in the brain alone; differences in the intensity of surgical stimulation can cause varying patterns of EEG changes. Furthermore EEG changes are dependent on the dose of anesthetic drug and vary among drugs, even drugs of the same class. In addition, hypothermia, hypoglycemia, hyponatremia, hypocarbia, and persistent hypoxemia can cause nonspecific slowing of EEG wave patterns. These pitfalls have combined to make observation of clinical signs still the only practical method of monitoring depth of anesthesia. (Although use of EEG to monitor anesthetic depth has remained an investigative tool, use of EEG and evoked potentials to monitor CNS function and surgical trespass is well established in neurosurgery and neurovascular surgery. The student should refer to specialized textbooks for these monitoring modalities.)

MONITORING CIRCULATORY FUNCTION

Pulse and Blood Pressure

It is customary to record the patient's pulse rate and blood pressure regularly at least every 5 minutes during the course of anesthesia. Such importance is placed on these variables because of the following considerations:

1. Pulse rate and blood pressure are time-honored vital signs.

2. Pulse rate and blood pressure, in addition to other clinical signs, are used as indicators of anesthesia depth (e.g., tachycardia and hypertension at levels inadequate for surgery; progressive hypotension at inappropriately deep levels).

3. Changes in pulse and blood pressure are recognized outcomes of certain surgical maneuvers or undesirable trespasses (e.g., bradycardia in response to traction on visceral organs or extraocular muscles; hypotension and tachycardia following hemorrhage).

4. Some anesthetic agents can alter cardiac rhythm, which may be evidenced by changes in the mechanical rhythm of the pulse (e.g., sinus or nodal bradycardia or cardiac standstill following succinylcholine).

Pulse rate, pulse volume, and mechanical rhythm of the heart can be obtained by palpation of an artery. In an emergency pulse volume may be used to estimate blood pressure. The radial pulse feels thready as blood pressure falls; it disappears when systolic blood pressure drops below 50 mm Hg; and the carotid or femoral pulse vanishes when systolic pressure drops to 30 mm Hg.

As an alternative to palpation, pulse can be monitored with a digital plethysmograph. Another method is auscultation using a mechanical or electronic precordial stethoscope positioned at the third interspace, just left of the sternum, or using an esophageal stethoscope placed at midsternal level. When heart sounds are monitored, loudness of aortic valve closure (the second sound) can be used as a semiquantitative index of diastolic pressure.

Sphygmomanometry by auscultation of Korotkoff's sounds in the upper arm is the traditional method of measuring blood pressure. When the upper extremity cannot be used, the cuff may be placed around the thigh. Accurate results are obtained only if the width of the cuff is approximately one-third the circumference of the arm or thigh. A cuff that is too narrow will give falsely high readings; one that is too wide will give spuriously low readings. If this method of sphygmomanometry is difficult (e.g., during hypotension or in obese patients), placement of an ultrasound flow transducer (the Doppler) over an artery distal to the cuff (e.g., the radial or dorsalis pedis artery) is a useful adjunct for measuring systolic blood pressure. (Systolic blood pressure is indicated by return of flow signals during deflation of the cuff.)

In the last decade, monitoring pulse rate and blood pressure by automated sphygmomanometers that operate on the principle of oscillometry has become commonplace. During their operation, pressure in the bladder of the cuff is automatically increased to above systolic pressure and then is decreased slowly in steps. At pressures between the systolic and diastolic range, pulsation in the partially obstructed artery is transmitted to the bladder. The amplitude of these pulsations is sensed by a transducer and its relationship to bladder pressure is analyzed by a microprocessor that computes systolic, diastolic, and mean blood pressure as well as pulse rate. These devices can be programmed to make repeated measurements at regular intervals—as frequently as every 20 seconds—and to sound an alarm when the measured variables fall outside chosen limits, but these instruments should not be abused. Too frequent determination of blood pressure using these devices has caused pressure injury to nerves. Measurements should not be made more frequently than every 5 minutes unless the patient's clinical condition warrants it.

Electrocardiogram

Continuous monitoring of the electrocardiogram (ECG) was originally introduced to monitor cardiac rhythm. Since the vector of lead II (right arm to left leg) parallels the P-wave axis, it is the most useful lead for monitoring electrical activities of the heart.

In recent years the ECG has also been recommended as a monitor of myocardial ischemia. A 1-mm horizontal depression of the S–T segment is accepted as a sign of subendocardial ischemia. Since more than 80% of ischemic changes occur in the left ventricle, precordial lead V_5 (left anterior axillary line at the fifth interspace) should be used for this purpose if it is available. If the electrocardiograph oscilloscope is equipped with bipolar leads only, modified precordial leads, CM_5 or CS_5, should be used. In the CM_5 modification the right-arm electrode of lead I is placed over the manubrium, the left-arm electrode over the V_5 position, and the ground electrode over the left shoulder. Lead CS_5 is similar to CM_5, except that the right-arm electrode is positioned over the right shoulder.

Invasive Hemodynamic Monitoring

Availability of plastic cannulas and catheters as well as transducers has made invasive hemodynamic monitoring simple. It allows continuous monitoring of arterial pressure, central venous pressure, and pulmonary capillary wedge pressure. The presence of these catheters also allows access for sampling of blood for arterial and mixed venous blood gas analysis.

Direct measurement of arterial pressure can be made via a cannula in a peripheral artery (radial, brachial, dorsalis pedis, common femoral, or left axillary); insertion of a 20-gauge cannula into the radial artery is the most popular method. Before this artery is cannulated, adequate collateral circulation from the ulnar artery should be demonstrated by the modified Allen's test: Occlude the radial and ulnar arteries with digital pressure while the patient clenches his fist. When the hand is exsanguinated, have him relax his fingers and hand in a neutral position. Adequate collateral circulation from the ulnar artery is confirmed by rapid capillary filling of the radial aspect of the hand when pressure on the ulnar artery alone is released.

Indications for the use of direct arterial pressure monitoring include the following:

1. Major cardiac, vascular, thoracic, and neurosurgical procedures
2. Other surgical procedures during which large fluid shifts are anticipated
3. Management of critically ill or high-risk patients
4. Cases in which blood pressure cannot be determined accurately using indirect methods
5. Use of "controlled hypotension" as part of the anesthetic technique

Central venous pressure can be measured with a catheter introduced into the superior vena cava via the internal jugular, external jugular, subclavian, or basilic vein. Measurement of central venous pressure is indicated when massive hemorrhage or fluid shift is anticipated. Individual values of central venous pressure are poor reflections of blood volume, but when the trend of these values and that of pulse rate, blood pressure, and urine output are considered together, central venous pressure measurement is an invaluable guide to fluid replacement. (Normal values for patients lying supine are 0–10 cm H_2O from the anterior axillary line or 4–14 cm H_2O) from the mid-axillary line.)

Measurement of *pulmonary capillary wedge pressure* (a reflection of left atrial pressure) has been popularized by introduction of the flow-directed Swan-Ganz catheter. A triple-lumen version of this catheter with a thermistor near its tip is available for measurement of *cardiac output* by thermal dilution; another version has an optical fiber incorporated into its lumen for continuous monitoring of *mixed venous oxygen saturation*. Measurements of pulmonary capillary wedge pressure and cardiac output are generally indicated during cardiac, major vascular, and major neurosurgical operations, in surgical patients with severe heart disease, and in those who are gravely ill.

MEASUREMENT OF BLOOD LOSS

The topic of blood transfusion to replace loss beyond a certain limit is discussed in Chapter 21. Unfortunately neither hemoglobin concentration nor hematocrit reflects the amount of blood loss during acute hemorrhage. The most simple and accurate method of measuring blood loss is to weigh discarded sponges and to measure the volume of blood in the suction apparatus. The difference in weight between blood-soaked and dry sponges in grams is equal to the volume of blood in the sponges in milliliters; the difference in volumes between fluid in the suction apparatus and irrigation fluid used is equal to the volume of blood removed by suction. Volume of blood spilled on surgical drapes is more difficult to measure, but with experience, the amount can be estimated with fair accuracy by careful inspection.

MONITORING RESPIRATORY FUNCTION

Clinical Signs

Invaluable information about the patient's respiratory function can be obtained by observing the respiratory rate, movement of the chest wall and abdomen, and excursion of the reservoir bag. The anesthetized patient who is not in distress breathes quietly. His chest wall rises and falls in rhythm with the reservoir bag, and his respiratory pattern is regular in both depth and rate. Irregular breathing or breath holding indicates inadequate anesthesia; a slow respiratory rate or apnea indicates overdose of opiates or other respiratory depressants. Paradoxical movement of the chest wall and abdomen, suprasternal in-drawing, and tracheal tug (downward movement of the thyroid cartilage with each inspiratory effort), with or without stridor, are pathognomonic for upper airway obstruction. Unequal movement of the two sides of the thoracic cage during inspiration is a sign of endobronchial intubation.

Clues to the adequacy of oxygenation and carbon dioxide elimination can be obtained by observing the patient's pulse rate, blood pressure, and color. Both hypoxemia and hypercapnia can cause tachycardia and hypertension; cyanosis is seen when more than 5 g of deoxyhemoglobin is present in each 100 ml of blood; a warm, flushed, moist skin is associated with hypercapnia. However, it must be stressed that the cardiovascular response to hypoxemia and hypercapnia is attenuated by anesthesia, and cyanosis may not be a reliable sign owing to the presence of natural pigmentation, poor lighting conditions, and cutaneous vasoconstriction. These are late signs that demand prompt action.

Ventilatory Volumes

During spontaneous ventilation, ventilatory function in healthy patients is usually judged by clinical signs alone, and ventilatory volumes are seldom measured routinely. During controlled ventilation, the bellows of the ventilator is usually calibrated to indicate inspired tidal volume. When independent verification is warranted during spontaneous or controlled ventilation, expiratory tidal and minute volumes can be measured by spirometry using mechanical devices, the most pouplar versions being the Wright respirometer and Dräger volumeter.

In the Wright respirometer gas flow is directed by a series of slots onto rotating vanes, and flow over time is registered as volume on a dial by the movement of a needle connected to the vanes by mechanical gears (Fig. 14–1A, B). It is basically a flow-sensing device designed for flow rates between 3 and 300 L/min. For accuracy, it is imperative to check that the vanes are free of water condensate before use. The Dräger volumeter is a similar device, but the flow-sensing mechanism is a pair of cogs that rotate in opposite directions (Fig. 14–1C). Again flow over time is transcribed by internal gears into movement of a needle on a dial. Both devices underestimate volumes in low flow conditions and overestimate when flow rate is high.

Airway Pressure

Airway pressure can be measured by incorporating an aneroid pressure gauge into the anesthetic circuit. It fluctuates around zero during spontaneous ventilation and seldom exceeds 30 cm H_2O at its peak during positive-pressure ventilation. Monitoring airway pressure is important in both instances. During spontaneous ventilation, positive pressure in the airway usually indicates that the

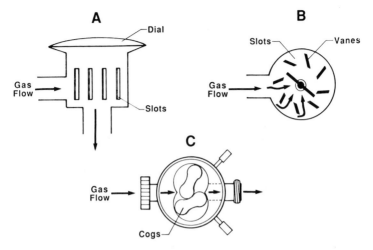

FIGURE 14–1. Wright respirometer: side view, *A*; cross-sectional view, *B*; and Dräger volumeter, *C*.

relief valve is not fully open (see "Relief Valve" in Chap. 8). During controlled ventilation, an increase in peak inspiratory pressure may mean an increase in airway resistance (e.g., bronchospasm, kinked endotracheal tube) or a decrease in pulmonary compliance (e.g., pulmonary congestion). A large drop in peak inspiratory pressure to below normal values during positive-pressure ventilation, on the other hand, always means a major leak in the circuit or complete disconnection. Current standards require that a low-airway-pressure alarm be incorporated into the breathing circuit during positive-pressure ventilation, to alert the anesthesiologist in case of such a disconnection (see "Pressure Gauge and Pressure Alarm" in Chap. 9).

Blood Gas Analysis

Information on *arterial O_2 and CO_2 tensions* (PaO_2 and $PaCO_2$), *pH,* and *buffering capacity* of arterial blood can be obtained by blood gas analysis. Normal PaO_2 is 95 mm Hg, but it can be as low as 70 mm Hg in healthy geriatric patients. Normal $PaCO_2$ is 35–45 mm Hg; normal arterial pH, 7.35–7.45; and normal standard bicarbonate concentration, 22–26 mEq/L. In general, blood gas analysis should be done at regular intervals during long procedures, in patients with cardiopulmonary disease, in seriously ill or severely injured patients, and during cardiovascular, intracranial, or thoracic operations. It must be stressed that blood gas analysis does not constitute continuous monitoring, even if it is done frequently, because results are always delayed and reflect past events. Intravascular electrodes with a rapid response time are available but require improvements before they can be recommended for general use.

Measurement of *transcutaneous oxygen tension* (tcPO$_2$) has been exploited as a noninvasive means of continuously monitoring oxygenation. In this method vasodilation and arterialization of subepidermal capillary blood is produced by heat, and oxygen diffusing through the epidermis is measured by a polarographic oxygen analyzer (see "Galvanic Fuel Cell and Polarographic Oxygen Analyzer," below.) Although tcPO$_2$ approaches PaO$_2$ when it is measured with meticulous care, its accuracy suffers when vasodilation is less than maximal (e.g., in low cardiac output states), when the epidermis is thick, and when oxygen consumption of surrounding tissue is high. Its application is more popular among infants and young children than among adults.

Another alternative to monitoring oxygenation is noninvasive measurement of arterial oxygen saturation (SaO$_2$) by *pulse oximetry*. This method is based on the differential absorption of red and infrared light by oxyhemoglobin and deoxyhemoglobin (Fig. 14–2A). While red light of wavelength 660 nm is absorbed strongly by deoxyhemoglobin and weakly by oxyhemoglobin, this difference is much less with infrared light of wavelength 940 nm. Light-emitting diodes (LEDs) in the pulse oximeter probe send light of these wavelengths through the test site (e.g., finger, earlobe, palm

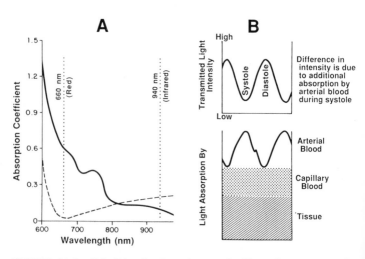

FIGURE 14–2. Principle of pulse oximetry. *A,* Absorption spectrum of oxyhemoglobin (*broken line*) and deoxyhemoglobin (*solid line*); *B,* pulsatile variation in light absorption by arterial blood.

of neonates) and the intensities of transmitted lights are monitored by sensors continuously. During diastole part of the incident light of both wavelengths is absorbed by a constant amount of tissue and blood in nonpulsatile capillaries (Fig. 14–2B). During systole the pulse-added portion of arterial blood absorbs additional light. At the peak of the pulse, these additional absorptions (equal to the difference between the intensity of transmitted light at the trough and that at the peak of the pulse) are related to the concentrations of oxyhemoglobin and deoxyhemoglobin in arterial blood alone. This difference in intensities is sensed by the photodetectors and fed into a microprocessor, which computes SaO_2 empirically.

$$SaO_2\% = \frac{\text{oxyHb conc}}{\text{oxyHb conc} + \text{deoxyHb conc}} \times 100\%$$

In addition, a pulse oximeter can act as a pulse plethysmograph and reproduce pulse wave forms on a monitor screen. Between saturation values of 60 and 100%, pulse oximeter measurements are accurate to ± 2.5%. But since other species of hemoglobin (carboxyhemoglobin, methemoglobin, sulfhemoglobin) have been ignored in the computation, the presence of a significant amount of abnormal hemoglobins in the patient's blood can yield erroneously high values of SaO_2. Although normal skin pigments do not interfere with measurement, the presence of bilirubin or dyes such as methylene blue and indocyanine green can produce errors. For accuracy the probe and test site must be protected from excessive movement and shielded from bright ambient lights, particularly infrared heat lamps, which are used on infants and young children.

MONITORING RESPIRATORY AND ANESTHETIC GASES

In order to protect the patient from exposure to hypoxic gas mixtures, anesthetic machines are equipped with an oxygen failure safety valve and alarm (see Chap. 7). For similar reasons continuous monitoring of inspired oxygen concentration has become a standard practice. Earlier models of these devices were based on galvanic fuel cell or polarographic principles; they had a slow response time and were suitable for monitoring only oxygen concentration in the anesthetic circuit. Monitors capable of measuring breath-to-breath concentrations of respiratory and anesthetic gases or vapors at the airway soon followed. They include paramagnetic oxygen analyzers, capnographs, nitrous oxide and halogenated vapor monitors, mass spectrometers, and Raman photospectrometers.

Galvanic Fuel Cell and Polarographic Oxygen Analyzers

The galvanic fuel cell oxygen analyzer is an electrochemical device consisting of one gold and one lead electrode immersed in a cesium hydroxide bath and separated from the gas sample by a semipermeable membrane (Fig. 14–3A). As it diffuses into the bath, each oxygen molecule combines with 4 electrons from the gold cathode and water molecules to form hydroxyl ions:

$$O_2 + 2H_2O + 4e^- \rightarrow 4OH^-$$

In turn these hydroxyl ions migrate toward the lead anode and react with it to form lead oxide and water, surrendering 4 electrons in the process:

$$4OH^- + Pb \rightarrow PbO_2 + 2H_2O + 4e^-$$

Constant diffusion of oxygen into the bath would mean a constant flow of electrons between the gold and lead electrodes and build-up of a potential difference that can be measured on a meter as oxygen concentration.

The polarographic (Clark-type electrode) oxygen analyzer is similar to the fuel cell model, but the silver-silver chloride and platinum electrodes are kept polarized with the help of a battery (Fig. 14–3B). Negatively charged hydroxyl ions formed by oxygen diffusing across the membrane are actively attracted toward the

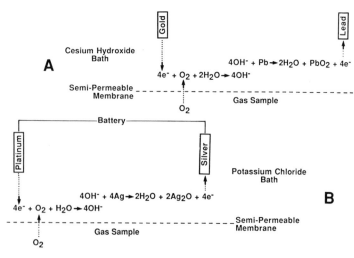

FIGURE 14–3. Principle of galvanic fuel cell oxygen analyzer, *A*, and polarographic oxygen analyzer, *B*.

positively charged silver-silver chloride electrode, thus improving the response time of this device. Nevertheless both the fuel cell and polarographic analyzers are designed for monitoring oxygen concentration in the anesthetic circuit only; their relatively slow response time precludes use for breath-to-breath measurement.

In order to make them true monitors, these instruments are equipped with low concentration alarms that warn the operator when oxygen concentration falls below a chosen limit. Common sense dictates that the lower limit should be set no lower than 21%. Since water condensate on the semipermeable membrane can interfere with oxygen diffusion, these sensors should be positioned at the fresh gas outlet of the anesthetic machine or at the inspiratory limb of the circle system proximal to the mouthpiece. Two-point calibration, at 21% and 100% oxygen, must be performed on these instruments daily before use.

Paramagnetic Oxygen Analyzers

Unlike other gases, oxygen is paramagnetic—that is, it has magnet-like properties. When exposed to a strong magnet, oxygen molecules align with and enhance the applied magnetic field. In the paramagnetic oxygen analyzer, dehumidified test sample and reference gas of known oxygen concentration (room air) are fed through tubing into adjacent test chambers between the two poles of an electromagnet that is being switched on and off repeatedly at a frequency of 110 Hz (Fig. 14–4A). Since forces acting on oxygen molecules in the on again-off again magnetic field will vary according to their concentration, an alternating pressure difference is generated between the test and reference chambers. This pressure difference is sensed by a differential pressure transducer, the signals are fed into a microprocessor, and oxygen concentration in the test sample is computed and displayed. Paramagnetic oxygen analyzers have a response time on the order of 200 msec and are capable of breath-to-breath measurement of inspiratory and expiratory oxygen concentration at the airway.

Capnographs

These devices measure instantaneous changes in CO_2 tension or concentration at the airway using infrared light absorption technology. A dehumidified test sample is drawn into a test chamber lying next to a reference chamber containing air, and identical beams of infrared light from an incandescent lamp are shined through both (Fig. 14–4B). After passing through these chambers, the two beams are filtered to allow only a narrow band of light with wavelengths around 4.3 μm to go through. Infrared light of this wavelength is strongly absorbed by CO_2. The difference in intensities of these filtered beams is directly related to the differ-

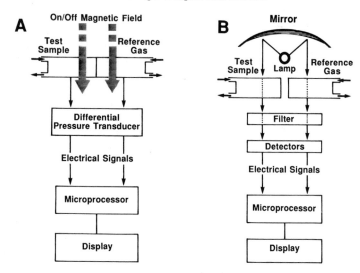

FIGURE 14–4. Diagrammatic illustration of paramagnetic oxygen analyzer, *A*, and capnograph, *B*.

ence in CO_2 concentrations between test sample and reference gas. This difference in intensities is sensed by infrared sensors, the signals are processed, and instantaneous CO_2 tension or concentration is displayed graphically on a monitor screen. With mainstream devices, the sensor is positioned close to the airway in line with the anesthetic circuit and response time is almost instantaneous (about 10 msec). With sidestream devices, test samples are withdrawn continuously from the airway via a pilot line and directed to a distantly located sensor. In this instance response time is dependent on the length of the pilot line and the rate of sample flow (usually around 150 msec).

Three major landmarks can be identified on a normal airway CO_2 wave form (Fig. 14–5*A*): an *inspiratory phase* and an *expiratory slope,* which rises rapidly to a well-developed *end-tidal plateau.* Since there is almost no alveolar-arterial CO_2 gradient in healthy subjects, end-tidal carbon dioxide ($ETCO_2$) level approximates arterial CO_2 tension of 35–45 mm Hg. But if development of the $ETCO_2$ plateau is cut off prematurely, as in tachypnea or bronchospasm (Fig. 14–5*B*), peak CO_2 levels in these instances are less than $ETCO_2$ values.

Inspiratory and $ETCO_2$ values and the shape of the wave form yield many clues to the functional status of the patient, the adequacy of ventilation, and the integrity of the anesthetic circuit.

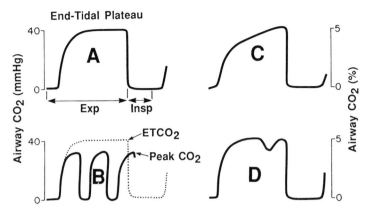

FIGURE 14–5. Airway CO_2 wave forms. *A*, Normal wave form; *B*, difference between peak CO_2 level during tachypnea and normal end-tidal CO_2 level during a normal breath; *C*, airway CO_2 wave form during partial airway obstruction; *D*, spontaneous tidal breath showed up as indentation of the end-tidal plateau of a ventilated breath.

(Capnometers that do not display an airway CO_2 waveform are not as versatile as capnographs.) During inspiration CO_2 tension of the inspired gas mixture should be near zero. If it is elevated to any degree immediate investigation and correction are imperative. Common causes of CO_2 appearing in the inspired gas mixture when the circle system is in use are (1) exhaustion of CO_2 absorption canister, (2) unintentional switching off of the canister, and (3) leak or backflow in unidirectional valves. When the Bain, Magill, or T-piece circuit is in use, the cause is always inadequate fresh gas flow.

In the absence of CO_2 rebreathing, $ETCO_2$ values depend on (1) adequacy of alveolar ventilation, (2) CO_2 production, and (3) state of pulmonary circulation. Proper interpretation of $ETCO_2$ values in anesthetized patients requires an awareness of the mode of ventilation and the trend of development of these values:

1. A mild degree of hypercapnia ($ETCO_2$ up to 60 mm Hg) during spontaneous ventilation is usually due to central respiratory depression by anesthetic drugs.

2. Gradual development of hypercapnia during controlled mechanical ventilation should raise the possibility of alveolar hypoventilation, a result of either inappropriate ventilator settings or leaks in the system.

3. Rapid development of hypercapnia during adequate mechan-

ical ventilation is associated with excessive CO_2 production in hypermetabolic states (e.g., hyperthermic crisis or thyroid storm). Checking the patient's body temperature and acid-base status and reviewing his medical history will help to clarify these issues.

4. Sudden development of hypercapnia during intra-abdominal CO_2 insufflation (e.g., in laparoscopic surgery) means CO_2 embolism.

5. A mild degree of hypocapnia during controlled ventilation is usually due to alveolar hyperventilation. If hypocapnia is inappropriate, hypometabolic states (e.g., inadvertent hypothermia and hypothyroidism) or large drops in cardiac output (e.g., hypovolemia and acute myocardial infarction) should be considered. In the former, CO_2 production is reduced; in the latter, diminished pulmonary perfusion leads to increases in physiologic dead space and arterial-alveolar CO_2 tension gradient.

6. Sudden and unexpected falls in ETCO$_2$ should raise the possibility of mechanical obstruction to the pulmonary circulation, as in pulmonary embolism (blood clot, air, amniotic fluid) or cardiac arrest.

In addition to inspired and end-tidal CO_2 values, the airway CO_2 wave form can be used as a diagnostic tool. In partial airway obstruction (e.g., bronchospasm or kinked endotracheal tube), the latter half of the expiratory slope rises slowly and continuously to merge with an ill-defined plateau (Fig. 14–5C). Partial recovery from muscle relaxants during mechanical ventilation may show up as indentations in the end-tidal plateau due to spontaneous respiratory efforts (Fig. 14–5D). Total disconnection during controlled ventilation is characterized by sudden disappearance of the wave form, and esophageal intubation by absence of the wave form following an assisted breath.

Nitrous Oxide and Anesthetic Vapor Monitors

Like capnographs these monitors are based on infrared light absorption technology. Nitrous oxide strongly absorbs infrared light in a narrow band around 3.9 μm; the filters in nitrous oxide monitors are adjusted to this band width, accordingly.

When it is applied to measuring anesthetic vapor concentrations, the operative infrared light absorption wavelength of 3.3 μm is not specific for the three halogenated volatile agents (halothane, enflurane, and isoflurane). These halometers cannot be relied on to distinguish one agent from another; they cannot recognize inadvertent admixture or substitution of agents. Unless the operator selects the correct setting for the agent in use, the displayed concentration is erroneous.

Mass Spectrometers

These instruments can distinguish and measure the concentration of all respiratory, anesthetic, and atmospheric gases and vapors. The test sample is injected into an ionization chamber, where all gas molecules become ionized through bombardment by electrons (Fig. 14–6A). The ionized molecules are then propelled through a magnetic field in the test chamber, in which each molecular species will follow a unique circular path depending on its charge-to-molecular weight ratio. These ion flows are registered as electric currents by sensors on the collecting plate, and the concentration of a gas is computed according to the following formulas:

$$\text{Total current} = O_2 \text{ current} + N_2O \text{ current} + CO_2 \text{ current} + \text{others}$$

$$O_2\% = (O_2 \text{ current/total current}) \times 100\%$$

Mass spectrometers have a response time of the order of 60 msec and can be used to monitor breath-to-breath inspiratory and end-tidal concentrations. Because they can measure nitrogen concentration, these devices have unique applications not available to dedicated monitors described previously:

1. End-tidal nitrogen concentration can be used to follow denitrogenation of the lungs during preoxygenation before rapid-

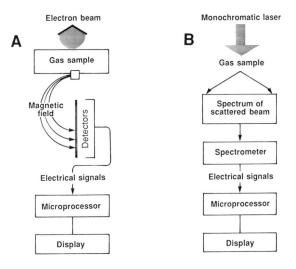

FIGURE 14–6. Diagrammatic illustration of mass spectrometer, *A*, and photospectrometer, *B*.

sequence induction (see "Rapid-Sequence Induction" in Chap. 15).

2. After denitrogenation is complete, the reappearance of end-tidal nitrogen is a sensitive indicator of air embolism.

3. Once nitrogen has been eliminated, reappearance of nitrogen during inspiration means the presence of an air leak.

All mass spectrometers in use today work on a time-shared basis between multiple locations. Depending on the number of locations in operation, intervals between sampling at any one location can vary from 1 to 5 minutes. That is, monitoring is intermittent rather than continuous; mishap and harm to the patient can occur without warning between samples. Dedicated single-user units will eliminate this danger.

Raman Photospectrometers

Like mass spectrometers, Raman photospectrometers can measure the concentration of all respiratory, anesthetic, and atmospheric gases and vapors. In these instruments a monochromatic (single wavelength) visible laser beam is directed at and scattered by molecules in the gas sample (Fig. 14–6B). Some of the photons (light particles) of the incident beam continue on without change in wavelength, and some emerge at different wavelengths, having gained energy from or lost it to the scattering molecules. Thus the emergent beam acquires a spectrum of wavelengths that is unique to the composition of the gas sample. Spectral analysis of the scattered beam is used to determine the concentration of each component.

MONITORING RENAL FUNCTION

Kidneys with normal concentrating function can excrete their daily solute load in as little as 600 ml of urine, but this is possible only if renal blood flow is normal. In general, a minimal hourly urine output of 25 ml is accepted as a sign of normal renal blood flow. Moreover, the ability of the kidneys to maintain this minimal hourly output has also been regarded as a sign of normovolemia and normal cardiac output. It is customary to monitor urine output via an indwelling urinary catheter when large fluid shifts or blood loss is anticipated during surgical procedures. Unfortunately opioids and stress can stimulate the secretion of antidiuretic hormone; and oliguria alone is not a reliable sign of hypovolemia or low cardiac output during surgery. A rational interpretation of urinary output can be made only if hemodynamic variables (pulse rate, blood pressure, and central venous pressure) and volume of blood lost during the operation are also taken into consideration.

MONITORING NEUROMUSCULAR FUNCTION

The popularity of muscle relaxants in current anesthesia practice has made it necessary to monitor neuromuscular function whenever these agents are used. Although clinical signs are helpful, an objective evaluation can be made only by using the peripheral nerve stimulator.

Clinical Signs

During abdominal surgery, a quiet operative field is a reliable sign of adequate muscle relaxation. Twitching of the diaphragm, appearance of bowel at the edge of the surgical wound, and appearance of skeletal muscle myopotentials on the electrocardiograph oscilloscope are indications for an additional dose of muscle relaxant.

At the end of the operation, return of neuromuscular function is signaled by the onset of spontaneous ventilation. The signs of adequate tidal exchange are quiet respiration, normal respiratory excursions that involve the apical regions of the chest wall, and absence of tracheal tug; however, they do not necessarily mean full recovery of neuromuscular function. The ability of the patient to exhale a vital capacity of at least 15 ml/kg, to generate a negative pressure of at least -25 cm H_2O on inspiration, to protrude the tongue, to lift the head off the pillow for 5 seconds, and to maintain a powerful hand grip are more helpful signs, but these tests are possible only when the patient is awake and can obey commands. Thrashing movements of the extremities and the trunk (like those of a "fish out of water"), inspiratory stridor, and muted coughs are signs of partial paralysis.

Peripheral Nerve Stimulation

Apnea may be due to central respiratory depression rather than paralysis, and the patient who is partially paralyzed may have an adequate tidal volume but will not be able to cope with increases in demand. In these situations, objective evidence of normal neuromuscular function should be sought by electrical stimulation of the ulnar nerve. Stimulation of the facial or lateral popliteal nerve has been used also for convenience. Many anesthesiologists advocate routine use of the peripheral nerve stimulator as an adjunct to observation of clinical signs whenever muscle relaxants are employed.

The peripheral nerve stimulator is designed to deliver a supramaximal electrical stimulus, which, when applied to a peripheral nerve, will elicit a muscle twitch. This stimulus can be delivered in three different modes: at a frequency of 1 Hz (single-twitch stimulus), at a frequency of 2 Hz for 2 seconds (train-of-4 stimulus), or at a frequency of 50 or 100 Hz (tetanic stimulus). The use of the peripheral nerve stimulator serves three purposes:

1. To differentiate the type of neuromuscular block
2. To determine the magnitude of the block
3. To determine the degree of recovery at the end of a procedure.

In the presence of a nondepolarizing neuromuscular block, stimulation of the ulnar nerve elicits the following motor responses in muscles of the hand (Fig. 14–7):

1. Lower-than-normal twitch height that fades gradually when the single-twitch stimulus is applied repeatedly
2. Similar fade in twitch height when the train-of-4 stimulus is applied
3. Unsustained response when the tetanic stimulus is applied
4. Transient increase in twitch response when the single-twitch stimulus is applied following tetany (a phenomenon called *post-tetanic facilitation*)
5. Disappearance of fade and of post-tetanic facilitation and return of twitch heights toward normal following administration of an adequate dose of anticholinesterase.

When a depolarizing muscle relaxant is used, the characteristic motor response to ulnar nerve stimulation during Phase I block is as follows (see Fig. 14–7):

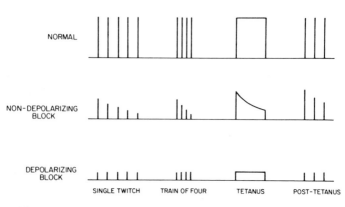

MONITORING DURING ANESTHESIA

FIGURE 14–7. Diagrammatic illustrations of muscle twitches in response to the electrical stimulation of a peripheral nerve.

1. Decreased twitch height that does not fade when the single-twitch stimulus is applied repeatedly
2. Absence of fade when the train-of-4 stimulus is applied
3. Tetany that is sustained
4. Absence of post-tetanic facilitation.

The characteristic response of Phase II depolarizing block is similar to that of nondepolarizing block.

It must be stressed at this point that these responses are seen only in the presence of partial blockade. When neuromuscular blockade is complete, no twitch response is seen; however, complete neuromuscular blockade is rarely necessary in anesthesia practice. A 90% reduction in single-twitch height is adequate for most abdominal procedures, and a reduction in twitch height of only 70% is required when an inhalation agent with muscle-relaxant action (i.e., enflurane or isoflurane) is used concurrently.

Since its introduction in 1975, the train-of-4 stimulus has been used extensively as a semiquantitative method of determining the magnitude of nondepolarizing block. When only the last of the four twitches is abolished, the degree of blockade correlates with a 75% reduction in single-twitch height; when the last two twitches are not detectable, reduction in single-twitch height is 80%; and when the last three twitches are not observable, reduction is 90%. Neuromuscular blockade is complete or 100% only when all four twitches are abolished. This method of assessing neuromuscular blockade requires no recording instrument. By counting the number of twitches in the train-of-4 response, the degree of neuromuscular blockade can easily be ascertained. Uneventful reversal of nondepolarizing blocks with an anticholinergic agent can be expected when three or more twitches are present. Reversal of nondepolarizing block should not be regarded as adequate until all four twitches in the train-of-4 have returned and when the strength of the last twitch approximates that of the first. As a diagnostic test for adequacy of antagonizing nondepolarizing blocks, sustained contraction in response to 50 Hz tetanic stimulation is even more reliable than the train-of-4 stimulus, but the former procedure is painful and cannot be used in patients who have regained consciousness.

Data correlating degree of neuromuscular blockade and its reversal to twitch heights were obtained by stimulation of the ulnar nerve. In clinical practice stimulation of the facial nerve is often used for convenience to monitor neuromuscular blockade. It must be emphasized that facial muscles recover from nondepolarization blocks earlier than muscles of the hand. Recovery of twitch heights in facial muscles when the train-of-4 stimulus is applied does not guarantee similar recovery in muscles of the hand.

MONITORING BODY TEMPERATURE

Thermometry to detect changes in body temperature during anesthesia should be practiced routinely. Hypothermia is a common complication during the course of anesthesia and surgery, and the drop in body temperature can be particularly severe in infants and small children, in critically ill patients, and when large volumes of fluid or blood are given. Hyperthermia, on the other hand, is much less common. It usually occurs during febrile illness or when waterproof surgical drapes are used in infants and small children. An unexpected rise in core temperature following induction of anesthesia in a cool operating room should raise the possibility of malignant hyperthermia (see "Malignant Hyperthermia" in Chap. 16).

Temperature can be measured with thermistors or thermocouples at many sites: mid-esophagus, nasopharynx, rectum, axilla, tympanic membrane, and skin. Usually esophageal or nasopharyngeal probes are used to measure core temperature in adults, and rectal probes in infants.

MONITORING OTHER SYSTEMIC FUNCTIONS

Frequently it is necessary to monitor other physiologic variables during the perioperative period, owing either to existence of concurrent illness or to complications of surgery. Blood sugar concentration should be determined periodically in diabetic patients, and electrolytes as well as buffer base should be followed in critically ill patients or in those who have had large fluid and electrolyte shifts. Furthermore, the need to monitor hemoglobin concentration and coagulogram in patients who have received large volumes of stored blood should not be overlooked.

BASIC INTRAOPERATIVE MONITORING

To monitor is to observe for changes so that the practitioner can be forewarned. In this role, the anesthesiologist is the master monitor: absorbing information and correlating and integrating all input data before dispensing an appropriate response. Therefore *continuous presence of the anesthesiologist* at the patient's side throughout the course of the procedure is the first cardinal rule of monitoring. If a temporary absence is necessitated by extenuating circumstances (e.g., attendance at life-threatening emergency), the anesthesiologist should transfer his duty to a surrogate who has agreed to take on the responsibility. During transfer of duty, he should summarize for his colleague the patient's medical history and findings, mode of ventilation under anesthesia, dosage of drugs received, and progress to date. In the event that momentary absence from the patient's side is required (e.g., due to radiation hazards), the anesthesiologist should remain in visual contact with the patient and his monitors and should return to the patient's side as soon as conditions permit.

Obviously the choice of monitors should be appropriate for the patient's medical condition and his surgical operation. Nevertheless a minimum level of monitoring should be practiced during the course of anesthesia even if the subject is an ASA Class I patient undergoing a simple surgical procedure. Many institutions and national organizations have published guidelines on this topic. The Standards for Basic Intraoperative Monitoring recommended by the American Society of Anesthesiologists are reproduced in Appendix II. Compulsory monitoring of the following parameters and functions during all anesthetic procedures are emphasized by these guidelines:

1. Display cardiac rhythm continuously on *ECG*.

2. Record *blood pressure* and *heart rate* at least every 5 minutes and check circulatory function more frequently by palpation of the pulse, ausculation of the heart, or other instrumentation.

3. Monitor *ventilation, oxygenation,* and *depth of anesthesia* by clinical signs.

4. Measure *oxygen concentration* in the breathing circuit using an oxygen analyzer with alarm, and monitor oxygenation by pulse oximetry.

5. Detect *disconnection* in the anesthetic circuit during controlled ventilation using a low-pressure alarm or similar device.

In addition to these methods, it is the consensus of many anesthesiologists that the automated sphygmomanometer, capnograph, peripheral nerve stimulator, and electronic thermometer are indispensable. They have proved to be cost effective and will become standard tools as guidelines for basic monitoring evolve.

In summary, vigilance is the cornerstone of monitoring. Emphasis should not be placed on the measurement of a single variable. Changes in all measured variables should be correlated and examined in the perspective of the patient's clinical condition.

Techniques of General Anesthesia

There are four phases in all techniques of general anesthesia: induction, maintenance, emergence, and recovery. Each phase requires skill and attention to details. Meticulous preparation and planning should be part of each anesthetic procedure. A little time well spent in preparation will save anxiety afterward.

A PRACTICAL GUIDE TO PREPARATION

Preparation in the operating room before arrival of the patient should include the following steps:

1. Fill syringes with appropriate intravenous agents and label them clearly.

2. Check that endotracheal equipment is available and in working order (see "Techniques of Intubation" in Chap. 13); this is necessary even if endotracheal anesthesia has not been planned because tracheal intubation may be required if complications develop.

3. Check that the pharyngeal suction apparatus is available on demand.

4. Switch on, set up, and calibrate all monitors.

5. Inspect the anesthetic machine and check that it has a duplicate supply of both oxygen and nitrous oxide and that vaporizers are filled with the correct volatile agents.

6. Inspect the carbon dioxide absorption canister of the circle system. Change the content of the canister if the dye indicator indicates exhaustion of absorbency.

7. Inspect the anesthetic circuit, fill the reservoir bag with oxygen, shut off the relief valve, and occlude the outflow of the circuit—compression of the bag should generate at least 40 cm

H_2O of pressure without leaking. Investigate if necessary. (The vaporizers and carbon dioxide absorption canister should be switched on in turn during this step so that leaks through these components can be ruled out.)

8. Attach a face mask of appropriate size to the anesthetic circuit.

9. Inspect the mechanical ventilator and check that it can generate positive pressure during inspiration and that the automatic changeover mechanism between inspiration and expiration is functioning.

When the patient is in the operating room, his identity and the nature and site of the scheduled operation should be checked once more. This is the last chance to avoid disasters of mistaken identity and misdirected surgery. Before induction of anesthesia the anesthesiologist should establish a freely running intravenous infusion, attach all monitoring devices, and record baseline values.

INDUCTION OF ANESTHESIA

The phase of induction begins when the anesthetic is first given to the patient and ends when surgical anesthesia is established. The trachea is intubated during this phase if endotracheal anesthesia is planned.

Before commencing induction, it is important to ascertain that the patient is secure on the operating table and that the arms are well supported. With onset of anesthesia and loss of muscle tone, poorly supported arms can fall off the edge of the table, producing shoulder dislocation or traction injury of the brachial plexus. Such accidents are preventable.

Intravenous Induction

Of all the intravenous induction agents (see Chap. 2), thiopental is still by far the most popular, but the method of induction is similar for all of them. Only the method for thiopental is described below.

Although the median induction dose of thiopental is 5 mg/kg, there is a wide variation in the requirement among individual patients. Therefore its dose should be titrated against observed effects. It is good practice to administer a test dose of 2 ml before giving the full dose. Pain at the site of injection following the test dose suggests a leak into perivenous space; pain distal to the site of injection in the digits should raise the possibility of intra-arterial injection (an accident that is complicated by thrombosis and gangrene). In either case, position of the intravenous cannula should be checked.

When thiopental is used for induction, most patients experience a taste of onion or garlic before onset of anesthesia. Some patients may yawn or take a deep breath at this point, but the most reliable sign of loss of consciousness is loss of eyelash reflex (blinking in response to stroking of the eyelash).

Once unconsciousness is established, a nitrous oxide-oxygen mixture should be given via face mask. The concentration of nitrous oxide should not exceed 70%, and total fresh gas flow should be consistent with that recommended for the anesthetic circuit being used (see Chap. 8). A volatile agent (halothane, enflurane, or isoflurane) should be added, and its concentration increased in 0.5% increments to 2–3%, so that an anesthetic level of alveolar concentration can be achieved quickly (see "Alveolar Uptake" in Chap. 3). Once surgical anesthesia is established, the concentration of the volatile agent can be returned to lower levels for maintenance. Some patients become apneic following an induction dose of thiopental; if this is the case, ventilation should be assisted until spontaneous respiration returns.

It must be emphasized that patients are only lightly anesthetized during induction. Unnecessary stimulation (e.g., catheterization of urinary bladder, manipulation of limbs) will provoke laryngospasm. No procedure, no matter how minor, should be allowed until surgical anesthesia is established.

Inhalation Induction

Inhalation induction via face mask with halothane is both rapid and pleasant. Except for transient movement of the extremities, breath holding, nystagmus, and a divergent gaze, the second stage described for ether is not seen. At the beginning of the procedure, only oxygen or a nitrous oxide-oxygen mixture without halothane should be given. When the patient has become accustomed to breathing through the mask, halothane should be added in 0.5% increments until its concentration is 3–4%. The patient should be allowed to take three or four breaths before each increase in concentration. Too rapid an increase can induce coughing and laryngospasm.

Onset of surgical anesthesia is marked by disappearance of both nystagmus and divergent gaze, by mid-sized pupils that react to light, and by a breathing pattern that is regular in rate and depth. When this stage is reached, the concentration of halothane can be returned to lower levels for maintenance.

Both enflurane and isoflurane can be used to induce surgical anesthesia in the manner described for halothane. However enflurane is a more potent respiratory depressant than halothane, and isoflurane is rather pungent. These properties can make inhalation induction somewhat more difficult.

Tracheal Intubation

If endotracheal anesthesia is planned, the trachea should be intubated soon after unconsciousness is established. Intubation is usually facilitated by administration of succinylcholine, 1 mg/kg, intravenously (1.5–2 mg/kg if precurarization is practiced). After onset of paralysis, the lungs should be ventilated gently with 100% oxygen for approximately 1 minute. This measure is necessary to fill the lungs with oxygen so that the patient can tolerate apnea during intubation without developing hypoxemia. (The technique of tracheal intubation is described in Chap. 13.) After tracheal intubation, manual ventilation of the lungs should continue with a mixture of nitrous oxide, oxygen, and a volatile agent until adequate spontaneous respiration has returned.

Rapid-Sequence Induction

Rapid-sequence induction (crash induction) is a technique in which the trachea is intubated during induction of anesthesia without manual ventilation of the lungs with pure oxygen beforehand. It is designed to minimize the risk of aspiration pneumonitis and is indicated in all clinical situations that predispose the patient to regurgitation or vomiting (e.g., obesity, pregnancy, bowel obstruction, acute abdomen, hiatus hernia, emergency operations). During this procedure, the presence of an assistant is absolutely necessary. The technique is as follows:

1. Check the anesthetic machine, the anesthetic circuit, and endotracheal equipment as described earlier. Be prepared for unforeseen difficulties and have at hand a backup laryngoscope and endotracheal tubes of different sizes.

2. Turn on the pharyngeal suction apparatus, which should be easily accessible.

3. Have the patient breathe 100% oxygen at high flow from a form-fitting mask for 3–5 minutes before induction of anesthesia. If end-tidal gases are monitored by mass spectrometry, allow enough time for denitrogenation of the lungs so that end-tidal nitrogen tension is less than 150 mm Hg. (This period of preoxygenation will eliminate the necessity for manual ventilation of the lungs with oxygen following onset of paralysis.)

4. With due consideration given to the patient's size, age, and state of health, determine the ideal induction dose of thiopental. Give this dose and 1 mg/kg of succinylcholine in quick succession.

5. As soon as the patient has lost consciousness, have the assistant apply pressure to the cricoid cartilage and direct it posteriorly. (The cricoid cartilage is the only tracheal ring that is complete. Pressure directed posteriorly on this cartilage will compress the esophagus against the sixth cervical vertebra and prevent regurgitation of stomach contents into the larynx and pharynx. This procedure is often referred to as "Sellick's maneuver.")

6. Intubate the trachea at onset of paralysis.

7. Inflate the cuff of the endotracheal tube before pressure on the cricoid cartilage is released.

8. Check the position of the endotracheal tube, make any necessary adjustment, and secure it in place.

After tracheal intubation, the course of anesthesia can proceed as described earlier.

In addition to these basic steps, some anesthesiologists recommend other measures to minimize the risk of regurgitation and aspiration. These measures include positioning the patient in a head-up position to prevent regurgitation or in a head-down or left lateral position to prevent aspiration. Unfortunately none of these measures is foolproof and all can make intubation difficult. One popular measure is precurarization (see "Precurarization" in Chap. 5). Succinylcholine-induced muscle fasciculation can cause a large increase in intra-abdominal pressure. Pretreatment of the patient with 3–6 mg of *d*-tubocurarine (or an equivalent dose of another nondepolarizing agent) given 2–3 minutes before succinylcholine can abolish this fasciculation and reduce the risk of regurgitation. It should be remembered, however, that precurarization reduces the potency and delays the action of succinylcholine. In order to obtain maximal muscle relaxation for intubation, the succinylcholine dose should be increased to 1.5–2 mg/kg following precurarization.

Positioning the Patient on the Operating Table

Following induction of anesthesia, a change in the position of the patient may be required for the operation. Although the choice of intraoperative position is made by the surgeon, every member of the surgical team should play an active role in ensuring that the patient is secure on the table. Improper postures and support can cause injuries and cardiovascular instability. Certain precautions should routinely be followed in positioning patients:

1. Make sure that the eyes are shut and protected. Pressure against the eyeballs can cause retinal vein thrombosis and blindness.

2. Protect the elbows. Allowing them to lie unpadded against the edge of the table can cause ulnar nerve palsy.

3. Do not abduct the arms farther than 90 degrees. Excessive abduction can cause traction injury of the brachial plexus.

4. Flex both knees and hips simultaneously during movement to the lithotomy position to avoid causing traction injury to the sciatic nerve.

5. Protect the knees in the lithotomy position. Allowing the lateral aspect of the knee to rest unpadded against the lithotomy post can cause lateral popliteal nerve palsy.

6. Make sure that the abdomen is free if the patient is in the prone position. Pressure against the abdomen can obstruct venous return and restrict excursion of the diaphragm.

7. Monitor vital signs closely when a sudden change in posture is made. Such changes can cause venous pooling, interfere with cardiac output, and result in disconnection of the anesthetic circuit or inadvertent extubation.

8. Do not allow bare metal parts of the operating table to come into contact with the patient. Electric currents used for cauterization running through these high-resistance pathways can cause electrical burns.

MAINTENANCE

After the patient is properly positioned, the operation may commence. When the operation is concluded, the depth of anesthesia should be lightened and the patient should be allowed to emerge. The phase of maintenance refers to the period beginning with the onset of surgical anesthesia and ending with emergence. One or more drugs can be given to maintain unconsciousness, analgesia, and muscle relaxation during this period. Whether a patient should be allowed to breathe spontaneously or whether controlled ventilation should be used during this period is not always easy to judge. Indications for controlled ventilation include the following:

1. Procedures requiring profound muscle relaxation for surgical access

2. Use of the nitrous oxide-narcotic-relaxant technique of balanced anesthesia

3. Intraoperative positions that restrict the respiratory excursion of rib cage or diaphragm (e.g., prone, steep Trendelenburg tilt, jackknife)

4. Presence of cardiorespiratory disease or other severe systemic illness

5. Cases in which hyperventilation is desirable (e.g., to reduce intracranial pressure).

Aside from these indications, the chosen mode of ventilation is a matter of the anesthesiologist's preference. In general, healthy patients are allowed to breathe spontaneously during short procedures, provided profound muscle relaxation is not required.

Spontaneous Ventilation

With operations that require only a mild degree of muscle relaxation (e.g., operations on extremities and the head and neck), spontaneous ventilation is usually allowed. With this technique, a mixture of nitrous oxide and oxygen (usually in a 2:1 ratio) is given for basal anesthesia and analgesia, a volatile agent is added as an adjunct to maintain unconsciousness, and an opioid is given as analgesic supplement when required. Since the combined respiratory depressant effects of the volatile agent and opioid can cause apnea, narcotic analgesic should be given in small increments only.

As a result of ventilatory depression (see Chap. 10), hypercapnia is always a complication of this technique; however, in healthy patients the degree of hypercapnia is usually mild when the correct fresh gas flow is used.

Controlled Ventilation

A neuromuscular blocking drug is used whenever profound muscle relaxation is required. Frequently it is also used in the nitrous oxide-narcotic-relaxant technique, even when profound muscle relaxation is not required for the operation. When use of a muscle relaxant is part of the technique, the patient's trachea is always intubated and controlled ventilation is instituted. The choice of agent is usually governed by the duration of the operation. When duration of the operation is to be less than half an hour, succinylcholine given intermittently or as a continuous infusion is the agent of choice. When duration of the operation is to be well under an hour, succinylcholine given as described or atracurium, gallamine, or vecuronium given when necessary is suitable. When duration of the operation is to be an hour or longer, intermittent doses of *d*-tubocurarine, metocurine, or pancuronium are more appropriate. In addition to muscle relaxant, nitrous oxide and oxygen, together with a volatile anesthetic or a narcotic analgesic or both, should be given to maintain unconsciousness and analgesia.

It is important to avoid hypoventilation and hyperventilation during controlled ventilation. This can usually be achieved by using a fresh gas flow and ventilatory volume recommended for the anesthetic circuit being used (see Chap. 8).

Controlled ventilation also can be achieved without muscle relaxants by using a volatile agent that has good muscle-relaxant properties to supplement nitrous oxide. With the availability of enflurane and isoflurane, use of such agents has become popular in cases when controlled ventilation is indicated but profound muscle relaxation is not required.

EMERGENCE

At the conclusion of the anesthetic, the patient is allowed to emerge from the stage of surgical anesthesia. The emergence phase is different for patients who are breathing spontaneously and for those whose ventilation is controlled.

The patient who is breathing spontaneously will emerge from surgical anesthesia as soon as administration of nitrous oxide and volatile agent is discontinued. If intubation was performed, the endotracheal tube can be removed, with the precautions previously described (see "Extubation" in Chap. 13). Extubation can be done either while the patient is still in the plane of surgical anesthesia or after protective laryngeal reflex has returned. (If aspiration of stomach contents, blood, debris, or pus is a potential complication, extubation should always be delayed until gag and cough reflex have returned.) If extubation is done at the plane of surgical anesthesia, the patient will probably require assistance in maintaining a patent airway (see "Airway Obstruction" in Chap. 16) and should be turned to a lateral position to prevent aspiration. If extubation is done after laryngeal reflex has been regained, a phase of breath holding and coughing (which is to be avoided after procedures such as intraocular and intracranial surgery) is likely. Because extubation while the patient is in a semiconscious state can result in laryngospasm it should be avoided.

During emergence the patient who has received succinylcholine should be allowed to recover from muscle paralysis spontaneously; the patient who has received a nondepolarizing muscle relaxant should be given an anticholinesterase together with an anticholinergic agent (e.g., neostigmine 2.5 mg and atropine 1.2 mg). As soon as neuromuscular function returns and ventilation is adequate, the patient should be allowed to emerge, as described above. If a muscle relaxant has been given, it is important not to let the patient regain consciousness before neuromuscular function returns. The experience of being awake but paralyzed is extremely unpleasant.

A potential complication in all patients during emergence is *diffusion hypoxia,* resulting from dilution of alveolar oxygen content by the large amount of nitrous oxide leaving pulmonary capillary blood during this phase. It can be prevented by having the patient breathe pure oxygen at high flow for at least 2 minutes before he is allowed to breathe room air. The risk is also minimized if care is exercised to avoid hypoventilation and airway obstruction during this period.

At the end of the operation, the patient should be admitted to a postanesthesia recovery area for continuing observation and care. The recovery phase of anesthesia begins with admission of the patient to this area, and emergence continues into this phase. The management of the patient during recovery is discussed in Chapter 18.

Management of Complications During Anesthesia

There are several complications that are common or important during the course of anesthesia. Some are due to an inappropriate level of anesthesia; others are part of the side-effects of anesthetic drugs; and still others are complications of pre-existing illnesses. As long as the patient is under his care, the anesthesiologist must be prepared to cope with these events without delay.

RESPIRATORY COMPLICATIONS

Hypoxemia, with or without hypercapnia, is a consequence of all respiratory complications. Even a mild degree of hypoxemia has the potential to cause harm. Cyanosis is a late sign of impaired oxygenation seen only when more than 5 g of deoxyhemoglobin is present in each 100 ml of arterial blood. Poor lighting and increased skin pigmentation can make cyanosis even harder to detect. Observing the color of blood in the operation site instead of color of skin, although more sensitive, is a haphazard method of detecting arterial desaturation. Monitoring by pulse oximetry is by far the most reliable. In order to prevent hypoxemia, inspired oxygen concentration should always be increased when respiratory complications develop in a patient under anesthesia.

Coughing

Coughing is a protective reflex in response to irritants in the airway. It is a complication seen at light levels of anesthesia. Irritation may be caused by the vapor of a volatile agent, the pharyngeal airway, saliva or mucus, or even gastric contents. Treatment should be directed at removing the irritant. The concentration of volatile agents should be increased only gradually during induction; a pharyngeal airway should be inserted only when the level of anesthesia is appropriate; and fluid contents in the pharynx should be cleared by suction. If gastric fluid is suspected, tracheal intubation is indicated, and the patient should be examined for signs of aspiration (see also "Aspiration of Gastric Contents" in this chapter).

Breath Holding

Breath holding is seen not infrequently during inhalation induction. It may also be seen in patients who are breathing spontaneously during maintenance. During inhalation induction, breath holding is a transient phenomenon. During maintenance, breath holding, with or without laryngospasm, can occur when a painful stimulus is applied and the level of anesthesia is inadequate. Spontaneous respiration will return when the painful stimulus is withdrawn, but surgery should not be allowed to proceed until depth of anesthesia is increased. If breath holding persists, attempts should be made to ventilate the lungs manually, but care should be exercised not to inflate the stomach with overzealous efforts. Manual ventilation is usually successful if laryngospasm is absent. The management of breath-holding with laryngospasm is discussed later in this chapter.

Airway Obstruction

The most common cause of airway obstruction in an unconscious patient lying supine is the tongue falling backward to lie on the posterior pharyngeal wall. In addition to signs of airway obstruction discussed earlier (see "Monitoring Respiratory Function" in Chap. 14), snoring occurs during inspiration and grunting, during expiration. This problem is easily corrected by flexing the neck, extending the head, and supporting the angles of the jaw. In some cases placement of a pharyngeal airway (either oral or nasal) may be necessary, and if improvement does not follow, tracheal intubation is indicated.

Kinking or compression of the endotracheal tube can cause airway obstruction in the intubated patient. Presence of a kinked or compressed segment can be confirmed by direct inspection or digital exploration. Correction of the defect is usually simple. Using reinforced tubes eliminates this problem.

Obstruction of the distal lumen of the endotracheal tube by a herniated cuff is a rarer cause of airway obstruction in intubated patients. This problem should be suspected if a thin suction catheter cannot be passed beyond the end of the tube. Deflating the cuff should resolve the problem.

Laryngospasm

Normally the vocal cords move apart on inspiration. During laryngospasm the cords are fixed in apposition, resulting in respiratory obstruction. If laryngospasm is only partial, stridor is heard during inspiration; in addition, exaggerated activities of the diaphragm, in-drawing, tracheal tug, and paradoxical movements of the abdomen and chest wall may be noted. If laryngospasm is complete, no stridor is heard. If laryngospasm and breath holding are both present, there is neither respiratory movement nor stridor. Like coughing, laryngospasm may be precipitated by irritation of the airway. It may also be caused by surgical stimulation applied at a light level of anesthesia.

Prolonged spasm can result in asphyxiation. Treatment should be directed at removing irritation or withholding stimulation, improving ventilation and oxygenation, and increasing the depth of anesthesia. If laryngospasm is only partial, assisted ventilation is usually successful; the spasm resolves spontaneously when depth of anesthesia is increased. When laryngospasm is complete, vigorous attempts at assisted ventilation only inflate the stomach and, so, should be avoided. When laryngospasm persists and attempts at assisted ventilation fail, 0.5 mg/kg of succinylcholine should be given intravenously to induce muscle relaxation. When the cords are paralyzed, controlled ventilation should be instituted, and tracheal intubation may be indicated.

Hypoventilation

There are many reasons for hypoventilation during anesthesia, including respiratory depression by anesthetic drugs, inadequate recovery from muscle relaxants, and airway obstruction. The consequence of hypoventilation is carbon dioxide retention and hypercapnia. Hypercapnia can coexist with hypoxemia, but it also can exist alone if high inspired oxygen concentration is administered. An elevated end-tidal CO_2 by capnography is the most reliable sign of inadequate ventilation, but certain clinical signs are also helpful: warm, flushed, and moist skin, tachycardia and hypertension, and increased oozing in the surgical field. In addition, careful observation may detect other clinical signs associated with the underlying cause of hypoventilation (e.g., apnea following intravenous barbiturates, shallow breaths in patients receiving a volatile agent, slow respiratory rate in patients receiving an opioid, signs of partial paralysis, and signs of airway obstruction).

Severe hypoventilation is a potentially fatal emergency. The patient found hypoventilating should be given ventilatory assistance immediately, and the inspired atmosphere should be enriched with oxygen. When the emergency is brought under control, definitive treatment should be directed at eliminating the precipitating cause. Sometimes it is more appropriate to assist or control ventilation until the end of the operation, when the patient's ability to maintain adequate tidal exchange can be reassessed. In severe illness, sensitivity to the effects of anesthetics, opioids, or muscle relaxants may be increased and ventilatory support may be needed well into the postoperative period.

Bronchospasm

Many anesthetic agents (e.g., thiopental, morphine, d-tubocurarine) can release histamine from mast cells and trigger the onset of bronchospasm in patients with asthma or bronchitis. Both ketamine and halothane have bronchodilating properties and are agents of choice in these patients. Halothane is also useful in the treatment of mild bronchospasm, but intravenous aminophylline and nebulization of ventolin into the airway are indicated if the attack is severe.

Bronchospasm can also be precipitated in lightly anesthetized patients by noxious stimuli (e.g., tracheal intubation). The spasm will subside if depth of anesthesia is increased. Halothane is again a useful agent for this purpose.

Aspiration of gastric contents may be the cause of bronchospasm that develops when the patient is under anesthesia. Aspiration may go unrecognized at the time of the incident. When it is diagnosed, prompt attention is crucial (see "Aspiration of Gastric Contents" below).

CIRCULATORY COMPLICATIONS

Hypotension

It is not uncommon to see blood pressure fall by 10–15% following induction of anestehsia in healthy persons; also it is not unusual for anesthetized patients with cardiovascular disease (e.g., atherosclerosis or hypertension) to have markedly lower pressures during periods when they receive little surgical stimulation. In addition, many other factors can cause hypotension during the course of an operation: circulatory depression by anesthetic agents, hypovolemia, interference of venous return or cardiac output by surgical packings and retractors, cardiac arrhythmias, acute myocardial infarction, underlying organic heart disease, and anesthetic accidents (e.g., hypoxemia, excessive airway pressure, tension pneumothorax, and transfusion of mismatched blood). Perfusion of brain, heart, kidneys, and liver is reduced during profound hypotension. The absolute lower limit of blood pressure required to maintain prefusion of these organs varies according to the patient's physical status and health. In general, a fall in blood pressure greater than 20% should be investigated.

In the face of severe hypotension, decisive actions are called for. Inspired oxygen concentration should be increased immediately, and specific treatment should be directed at elimination of the underlying cause: decreasing the depth of anesthesia if possible; replacing volume deficit; rectifying mechanical interference of venous return or cardiac output; treating cardiac arrhythmias; ruling out acute myocardial infarction; draining pneumothorax; and treating mismatched transfusion. For severe myocardial disease circulatory support with an inotropic agent is indicated (e.g., dopamine, 5–50 μg/kg/min or dobutamine, 2.5–40 μg/kg/min).

Hypertension

Hypertension during anesthesia is as common as hypotension. It usually occurs as a response to noxious stimuli (e.g., tracheal intubation and traction on visceral organs) and is a sign of inadequate anesthesia. Other causes of intraoperative hypertension include hypercapnia and hypoxemia, pre-existing arterial hypertension, fluid overload, and undiagnosed and untreated pheochromocytoma.

The pressor response to tracheal intubation is preventable by increasing the depth of anesthesia, although this may not be appropriate in ill patients. An alternative is to apply lidocaine to the pharynx, larynx, and trachea before intubation or to administer lidocaine 1.5 mg/kg 1½–3 minutes before the procedure is attempted. The rise in blood pressure is also minimal if intubation is done gently, skillfully, and swiftly.

Hypertension in response to surgical stimulation should be treated either by increasing the concentration of the volatile agent or by an additional dose of an opioid. Patients with cardiovascular disease are prone not only to have low blood pressure during periods when stimulation is minimal but also to react to stimulation with a marked increased in blood pressure. Depth of anesthesia should be carefully monitored in these patients. As described earlier, hypertension may be secondary to hypercapnia or hypoxemia and should be treated accordingly.

Arrhythmias

The incidence of cardiac arrhythmias during anesthesia is extremely high, even in patients without organic heart disease. Arrhythmias may be precipitated by anesthetic agents in use or by manipulation during anesthetic and surgical procedures. Fortunately most of these disturbances are benign.

Sinus tachycardia following administration of atropine, pancuronium, gallamine, or ketamine is benign in patients without organic heart disease and requires no treatment. Sinus tachycardia in response to tracheal intubation or surgical stimulation is a sign of inadequate anesthesia and will disappear when depth of anesthesia is increased. Hypoxemia, hypercapnia, or hypovolemia can also cause sinus tachycardia and should be corrected promptly.

Atrial flutter or *fibrillation* is rare but always serious. The abnormality may be precipitated by manipulation of the heart during thoracic operations, particularly in geriatric patients and those with organic heart disease. In the operating room, atrial flutter or fibrillation of acute onset should be treated by direct-current cardioversion. If this is unsuccessful, digitalization may be necessary to control the ventricular rate.

A lower-than-normal heart rate is common in patients receiving halothane or large doses of morphine or fentanyl for maintenance. Treatment with atropine is not necessary, unless there is a concurrent fall in blood pressure. However, profound *bradycardia* and transient *asystole* require immediate attention. These disturbances are frequently associated with repeated doses of succinylcholine or traction on extraocular muscles. They can be prevented or treated with atropine, 0.6 mg, given intravenously.

A slow *nodal rhythm,* another common complication in patients receiving halothane for maintenance, is usually benign. However, sequential atrioventricular contraction can account for as much as 25% of stroke volume in a small number of patients. If nodal bradycardia causes hypotension, it should be treated with atropine.

A third rhythm disturbance often found in patients receiving halothane is *ventricular premature beats*. They are particularly common if hypercapnia is allowed to develop or if epinephrine is used to infiltrate the surgical field. Ventricular arrhythmias due to interaction of halothane and hypercapnia will disappear if $PaCO_2$ is returned to normal by increasing ventilation. Arrhythmias due to interaction of halothane and epinephrine, on the other hand, can be bizarre and alarming. Dose of epinephrine used to infiltrate the operative site should be limited to 10 ml of 1:100,000 concentration in 10 minutes or 30 ml in 1 hour. Lidocaine, 1 mg/kg or 30 μg/kg/min, may be necessary to treat ventricular premature beats that are frequent (more than 5 per minute), those that come in runs of three or more, those that are multifocal in origin, and those that fall on the T-wave of the preceding beat.

Patients who have organic heart disease, hypokalemia, or acidemia are more prone to develop serious arrhythmias during anesthesia. In these patients, careful evaluation should be carried out and the abnormalities should be treated in the preoperative period.

ASPIRATION OF GASTRIC CONTENTS

This is a potentially fatal complication of anesthesia. Patients who are at risk include those who have bowel obstruction, acute abdomen, or disease of the stomach or esophagus; those who are pregnant or obese; those who have sustained severe injuries; and those who require emergency operations. The consequences of aspiration vary according to the physical characteristics of the inhaled material. Solids, by obstructing the tracheobronchial tree, cause atelectasis. Gastric juice with a pH of less than 2.5 will cause acid pneumonitis (Mendelson's syndrome). Clinical signs of acid pneumonitis are cyanosis, tachycardia, tachypnea, rales, and rhonchi. In a florid case, signs of pulmonary edema and circulatory collapse may be seen. Whereas clinical signs of atelectasis are usually obvious immediately following aspiration of solids, those of acid pneumonitis may be delayed for several hours.

Aspiration pneumonitis is a preventable complication. In patients predisposed to regurgitation, the airway should be protected with a cuffed endotracheal tube. Use of the rapid-sequence induction technique and delay of extubation until return of laryngeal reflex are advised in these patients. Should aspiration occur, solids should be removed by bronchoscopy and liquids by postural drainage or trancheobronchial toilet. Some degree of pneumonitis occurs after any acid aspiration. The sequelae of a minor episode are usually mild and require only symptomatic treatment, but pulmonary edema and severe hypoxemia due to massive aspiration require intensive therapy.

The most effective means of improving arterial oxygenation following massive aspiration is to control ventilation and to apply positive end-expiratory pressure (PEEP). The level of PEEP should be adjusted to yield the best oxygenation without decreasing blood pressure or cardiac output. Since a large portion of the circulating volume may be lost as pulmonary edema fluid, aggressive replacement is indicated. Continuous measurement of arterial and central venous or pulmonary capillary wedge pressure, as well as intermittent sampling of arterial blood for blood gas analysis, is necessary to guide therapy. With optimal supportive care, the disease process is self-limiting and recovery is spontaneous. There is little indication that steroids will alter the course of acid pneumonitis. Antibiotics, on the other hand, should be used when there is evidence of secondary bacterial infection.

MALIGNANT HYPERTHERMIA

Malignant hyperthermia is caused by a rare skeletal muscle disease. The victims, usually children or young adults, are prone to develop life-threatening hyperpyrexia under anesthesia. There appears to be a large regional variation in the prevalence of this disease; incidence of malignant hyperthermic crisis has been reported to be as high as 1 in 20,000 anesthetic procedures and as low as 1 in 100,000. The syndrome is characterized by a hypermetabolic, hyperthermic state precipitated by succinylcholine and volatile anesthetics, and occasionally by physical or emotional stress. The pathologic mechanism is believed to be initiated by loss of control over calcium ion sequestration and reuptake in skeletal muscle fibers leading to contracture, increase in oxygen consumption, and increase in lactate and heat production.

Pedigrees of affected persons suggest that the trait is inherited either in an autosomal-dominant pattern with reduced penetrance and variable expressivity or in a multifactorial pattern involving more than one gene. Many patients who have the malignant hyperthermia trait have abnormal muscle morphology (excessive bulk), other skeletal muscle abnormalities (e.g., strabismus, inguinal hernia, club foot), cardiomyopathy, or elevated serum creatine kinase. All patients who are first-degree relatives of a person known to have had malignant hyperthermia or to have tested positive should be regarded as potential victims until proven otherwise; as should all members of an affected family who have skeletal muscle abnormalities or elevated serum creatine kinase. Contrary to previous belief masseter spasm or trismus, which occurs in 1% of children given succinylcholine against a background of halothane anesthesia, is not a sign of imminent hyperthermic crisis.

Muscle biopsy and determination in vitro of contracture response to caffeine and halothane is the only reliable diagnostic test for malignant hyperthermia to date. Serum creatine kinase level has no diagnostic value as a screening test in the general population. Nor does a normal serum creatine kinase level rule out susceptibility in members of a family known to have malignant hyperthermia. But elevated values in members of an affected family demand further investigation. Halothane-induced depletion of platelet ATP and calcium uptake by muscle strips have been suggested also as diagnostic tests but have been found to be unreliable. Currently three noninvasive tests are under investigation: (1) measurement of ankle torque and its modification by dantrolene, (2) halothane-induced changes in ionized calcium within lymphocytes, and (3) phosphorus nuclear magnetic resonance spectroscopy. Results are still pending.

All patients suspected to have the malignant hyperthermia trait should receive dantrolene for prophylaxis (1–2 mg/kg orally every 6 hours for 1–2 days, up to 3–5 hours before the operation and for 3 days after the operation). In addition, these patients should not be exposed to agents that can trigger a crisis, including all volatile agents and succinylcholine. Since only a trace of volatile anesthetic can precipitate an attack, an anesthetic machine without vaporizer reserved for this purpose should be employed. A machine that has been purged overnight with a high flow of oxygen after its vaporizers have been removed is also suitable. Similarly an uncontaminated anesthetic circuit and ventilator should be used.

Since inappropriate hypercapnia and hypoxemia are early signs, the capnograph and pulse oximeter have been recognized as the best monitors to give early warning of an impending crisis. Other signs of an attack include tachycardia, tachypnea, ventricular arrhythmia, muscle rigidity, cyanosis, mottled skin, profuse sweating, inappropriate increase in body temperature, arterial and mixed venous desaturation, respiratory and metabolic acidosis, electrolyte abnormalities, myoglobinemia, myoglobinuria, and elevated serum creatine kinase. Late complications include disseminated intravascular coagulation, renal failure, muscle necrosis, and coma. The mortality rate following an acute crisis is over 50%. Successful treatment depends on early recognition and intensive therapy. The onset of a crisis requires immediate institution of the following measures:

1. Stop administration of all offending agents.
2. Inform the surgeon and request that the operation be concluded as soon as possible.
3. Call for help to obtain central venous access, to cannulate an artery for blood samples and pressure monitoring, and to introduce an indwelling urinary catheter.
4. Hyperventilate the patient with 100% oxygen at a high rate of flow.
5. Administer dantrolene, 1 mg/kg, intravenously in a bolus. Repeat the dose if necessary until the total dose is 10 mg/kg. (Dantrolene can abort a crisis. Treatment with dantrolene, 1–2 mg/kg every 6 hours should be continued for 1–3 days after the crisis is arrested.)
6. Treat sinus tachycardia with propranolol and ventricular arrhythmias with procainamide (Procainamide, 15 mg/kg, given intravenously can abort an attack. Unfortunately it also can cause cardiotoxicity and hypotension.)
7. Treat hyperkalemia with glucose-insulin infusion at the initial stage, but be prepared to give potassium chloride intravenously at a later stage. (Potassium leaked out of skeletal muscle cells during the initial stage of a crisis can cause cardiac standstill. As the crisis subsides and diuresis is induced, hyperkalemia can give way to hypokalemia. Therefore frequent measurement of serum electrolyte contents is necessary.)
8. Correct respiratory and metabolic acidosis. (Sodium bicarbonate reacts with hydrogen ions to release more carbon dioxide and can cause hypernatremia and hyperosmolarity. The current

trend is to use sodium bicarbonate more conservatively than was previously recommended. Arterial pH will return toward normal when hypercapnia is corrected by hyperventilation. But if pH remains below 7.2, sodium bicarbonate should be given intravenously to correct metabolic acidosis according to the formula described under "Acid-Base Abnormalities" in Chap. 20.)

9. Induce diuresis when indicated. (Dantrolene preparation contains 3 g of mannitol per 20-mg vial, which is enough to induce a moderate degree of osmotic diuresis. If the patient is hypernatremic or if hyperkalemia persists, furosemide should be given intravenously to increase urinary excretion of sodium and potassium.)

10. Cool the patient if body temperature is 39° C or above. (Dantrolene has replaced cooling as the mainstay of treatment. Elevated body temperature will subside as dantrolene takes effect. Aggressive cooling is no longer recommended.)

In the event of a crisis, time is crucial in aborting an attack. Therefore all drugs and equipment mentioned above should be readily available before a potential victim is anesthetized. (At least thirty-six 20-mg vials of dantrolene should be available on site in institutions in which anesthesia is practiced.)

Techniques of Local and Regional Anesthesia

In skilled hands local and regional techniques provide excellent anesthesia for many surgical procedures. Although the systemic actions of local and general anesthetic agents are different, patients merit the same attention whether they are scheduled for local or for general anesthesia. General preoperative assessment should be performed, and it is also important to establish that these patients are willing subjects, that they do not have a history of bleeding diathesis, and that there is no infection at the site of injection. Pre-existing neurologic deficits should be regarded as a relative contraindication to nerve blocks and spinal or epidural anesthesia. Since most patients are anxious about being awake during the operation, an anxiolytic agent should be included in the premedication. In the operating room, a freely running intravenous infusion should be established, and equipment for resuscitation should be checked before major blocks are attempted. During the entire course of the operation, vital functions should be monitored.

Introduction of pathogenic organisms by needle is always a potential danger with all regional techniques. Therefore major regional blocks should be attempted only in a sterile setting: long hair at the site of injection should be shaved off; site of needle entry should be cleansed and draped; the anesthesiologist should wear cap, mask, and gloves; and sterile equipment should be used. Since injection of the anesthetic solution into intravascular space is a potential complication, thorough aspiration before injection is mandatory. In the sections that follow, some common techniques of local and regional anesthesia using lidocaine as an example are described. (Equivalent dose for other local anesthetic agents appears in Chap. 6.) Unless otherwise specified, use of a 22-gauge needle is appropriate in the following procedures.

LOCAL INFILTRATION

Local infiltration is suitable for suturing superficial wounds and excising cutaneous or subcutaneous lesions. Epinephrine may be added to prolong the action of the anesthetic agent in this technique, but its concentration must be limited to 1:200,000, because necrosis of skin edges is a potential complication.

The technique of local infiltration is as follows:

1. Pierce the skin with the needle and raise a wheal by injecting a small amount of 0.5% lidocaine.

2. Advance the needle to deposit more lidocaine on either side of and beneath the lesion (Fig. 17–1A).

3. Make subsequent entries with the needle at sites already anesthetized, and deposit more lidocaine solution until the lesion is encircled.

DIGITAL NERVE BLOCK

Each finger or toe is supplied by two dorsal and two palmar digital nerves alongside the digit. A digital nerve block is satisfactory for simple operations such as suturing wounds and excising nails. The technique of digital nerve block is as follows:

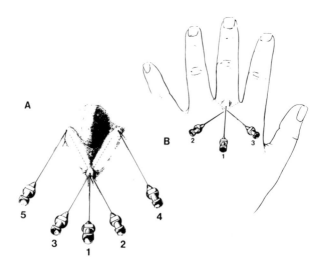

FIGURE 17–1. Techniques of local and regional anesthesia. *A*, Local infiltration. *B*, Digital nerve block.

1. Approach the digital nerves from the dorsal aspect of the hand or foot.

2. Raise a skin wheal close to the base of the digit (see Fig. 17–1B).

3. Advance the needle to deposit 1–1.5 ml of 1.5% lidocaine on both sides of the digit.

Injection of a large volume of anesthetic solution and addition of vasoconstrictor should be avoided in this technique. Both can compromise the circulation of the digit, either by mechanical compression or by constriction of the digital arteries.

INFILTRATION OF FRACTURE HEMATOMA

Both the periosteum and soft tissue at the site of a fracture can be anesthetized adequately by infiltrating the fracture hematoma. The technique is both simple and safe, and onset of anesthesia is usually obvious within 5 minutes. The technique is as follows:

1. Raise a skin wheal over the fracture site.

2. Advance the needle into the hematoma.

3. Verify the position of the needle by aspirating for blood.

4. Deposit 10–15 ml of 1.5% lidocaine without epinephrine in the hematoma. (The injection should be made slowly as rapid injection can cause pain.)

A major disadvantage of this technique is lack of muscle relaxation. It should be used only for closed reduction of simple fractures (e.g., Colles' fracture).

INTRAVENOUS REGIONAL ANESTHESIA

Intravenous regional anesthesia is a simple technique that provides excellent anesthesia and muscle relaxation for operations on the extremities. The technique is as follows:

1. Cannulate a peripheral vein on the limb to be anesthetized with a plastic cannula.

2. Exsanguinate the limb by simple elevation or by using an Esmarch bandage. (Proper exsanguination of the limb reduces the volume of anesthetic solution required.)

3. Place an arterial tourniquet around the arm or thigh and inflate it to a pressure of 100 mm Hg above the patient's systolic pressure.

4. Inject 0.6 ml/kg of 0.5% lidocaine without epinephrine intravenously via the indwelling cannula for anesthesia in an upper

extremity. Increase the volume to 1–1.2 ml/kg for a lower extremity.

5. Remove the venous cannula when anesthesia is established. (The onset of warmth and a tingling sensation should be immediate, and anesthesia should be complete within 15 minutes.)

A major limitation of this technique is the large dose of lidocaine required, particularly for the lower limbs. The arterial tourniquet should not be deflated for at least 15 minutes after injection of the local anesthetic solution; otherwise rapid uptake of lidocaine can cause systemic toxicity. Since sensation will return within 2–5 minutes following deflation of the tourniquet, a second limitation is restriction on the duration of the operation imposed by the maximal period of interrupted circulation considered safe (usually not more than 90 minutes). A third limitation is pain at the site of the tourniquet. Pain can be prevented by using the double tourniquet technique (Fig. 17–2), in which anesthesia is induced with the proximal cuff inflated. When discomfort develops at the site of this cuff, the distal cuff is inflated and the proximal cuff is deflated, in that order. Since the distal cuff lies over an anesthetized area, tourniquet pain is minimized.

BRACHIAL PLEXUS BLOCK

The brachial plexus arises from the anterior rami of spinal nerves C5–C8 and T1, with contributions from C4 and T2. These segmental nerves join to form trunks, divisions, and cords that emerge between the scalenus anterior and scalenus medius to lie between the clavicle and the first rib, lateral and posterior to the subclavian artery. In the axilla and beyond they divide to form

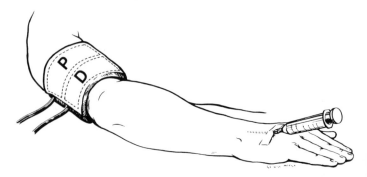

FIGURE 17–2. Intravenous regional anesthesia of the upper extremity using a double arterial tourniquet. The proximal cuff is *P*, and the distal cuff, *D*.

the major nerves supplying the arm and the forearm. Together with the subclavian artery and vein, the plexus is ensheathed in connective tissue to form the neurovascular bundle. Extensive surgery on the upper extremities can be done under a brachial plexus block.

Supraclavicular Approach

For brachial plexus block using the supraclavicular approach, anesthetic solution is deposited in the sheath of the neurovascular bundle as it crosses the first rib. The technique is as follows:

1. Position the patient supine with the arm by the side and the head turned to the opposite side.
2. Locate the subclavian artery and depress it with the index finger of one hand. (The artery can usually be located just behind the midpoint of the clavicle.)
3. Raise a skin wheal at this point and with the other hand advance the needle toward a site immediately behind the artery. Direct the needle mediad (toward midline), posteriorly (toward the patient's back), and caudad (toward the patient's foot) as illustrated in Figure 17–3A.
4. Inject 20–25 ml of 1.5% lidocaine with epinephrine into the neurovascular sheath. (Injection should be made only after paresthesia is elicited. If the needle touches the first rib, its tip is beyond the plexus; it should be withdrawn and redirected accordingly.)

A serious complication of supraclavicular brachial plexus block is pneumothorax. This problem should be suspected if the patient coughs while paresthesia is being sought, if air is aspirated during

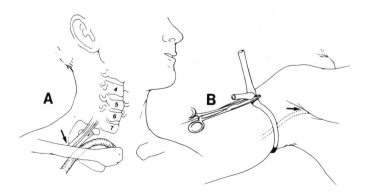

FIGURE 17–3. Brachial plexus block. *A*, Supraclavicular approach. *B*, Axillary approach.

advancement of the needle, or if the patient complains of respiratory distress. When the suspicion is confirmed, the patient's respiration should be monitored and the size of the pneumothorax assessed on chest x-ray films. A patient who has symptoms should be given oxygen by face mask. Drainage of the pleural space by an intercostal tube connected to an underwater seal may be necessary. Owing to the proximity of the phrenic nerve, the recurrent laryngeal nerve, and the stellate ganglion, paralysis of these nerves and Horner's syndrome are occasional complications.

Axillary Approach

Axillary approach to the brachial plexus block offers little or no anesthesia on the lateral aspect of the arm, but it is an excellent technique for use in operations on the hand, forearm, and elbow. The technique is as follows:

1. Position the patient supine with the arm abducted 90 degrees and externally rotated.

2. Apply a venous tourniquet to the arm just beyond the axilla, as shown in Figure 17–3*B*. (In some patients the musculocutaneous nerve leaves the lateral cord of the plexus high up in the axilla. The venous tourniquet helps to spread the anesthetic solution cephalad to include this nerve.)

3. Identify the axillary artery at the highest point in the axilla.

4. Raise a skin wheal at this point and advance the needle toward a site adjacent to the artery. (A click is felt by the operator as the needle punctures the neurovascular sheath, but the patient may or may not feel paresthesia.)

5. Inject 25–30 ml of 1.5% lidocaine with epinephrine into this neurovascular space.

The axillary route is a popular approach because there is no risk of pneumothorax. However the time of onset may be delayed for up to 30 minutes.

SPINAL ANESTHESIA

The spinal cord extends down to the second lumbar vertebra (L2) and the dural sac, to the second sacral vertebra (S2). Therefore the subarachnoid space between L2 and S2 contains only cerebrospinal fluid and lumbar and sacral nerve roots (the cauda equina). Local anesthetic solution deposited in the lumbar subarachnoid space can travel caudad and cephalad to provide anesthesia for operations on the perineum, the external genitalia, the lower extremities, and abdominal organs.

Dural puncture for spinal anesthesia requires both care and skill. The technique is as follows:

1. Position the patient on one side with the spine flexed.
2. Identify the L3–4 interspace on an imaginary line joining both iliac crests.
3. Raise a skin wheal at the center of the interspace.
4. Advance the spinal needle (22-gauge or smaller) with its stylet in place in a direction perpendicular to the skin but pointed slightly cephalad. Note the changes in resistance to advancement of the needle as it traverses the subcutaneous tissue, supraspinous ligament, interspinous ligament, ligamentum flavum, epidural space, and dura (Fig. 17–4). (A click can be felt as the dura is pierced, and the patient may complain of paresthesia in the lower extremities at the same time.)

The subarachnoid space is approximately 6 cm from the skin surface in a person of average build. If bone is encountered before the space is entered, the needle should be withdrawn, the landmarks redefined, and the needle redirected accordingly. Dural puncture at lower spaces may be successful when those at L3–4 fail. A clear flow of cerebrospinal fluid when the stylet is removed confirms that the tip of the needle is in the subarachnoid space. Persistent paresthesia and grossly bloody spinal fluid that does not clear are indications for readjusting the position of the needle. Local anesthetic should be injected only when there is free flow of clear spinal fluid.

The agent most commonly used for spinal anesthesia is tetracaine made hyperbaric by mixing a 2% solution with an equal volume of 10% dextrose. The dose of tetracaine is governed by

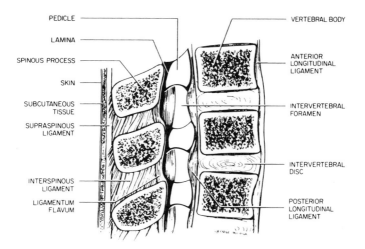

FIGURE 17–4. Sagittal section of the spinal canal with its contents removed.

the spinal level at which anesthesia is required. In a patient of average build 6 mg is required for operations on the perineum, 10 mg for operations on the external genitalia or the lower extremities, 12 mg for operations on the urinary bladder and the inguinal region, 14 mg for operations in the lower abdomen, and 16 mg for operations in the upper abdomen. Each of these doses should be reduced by 2 mg in shorter-than-average patients and increased by 2 mg in taller-than-average patients. After deposition of the local anesthetic, the needle is withdrawn and the patient is turned carefully to the supine position with hips and knees flexed and head resting comfortably on a pillow. Onset of anesthesia is rapid and is preceded by a feeling of warmth in the lower extremities. (The agent of choice in operations lasting less than 1½ hours is 5% hyperbaric lidocaine rather than tetracaine. On a weight-for-weight basis the dose of lidocaine should be increased by a factor of 5.)

Many factors other than dose can increase the number of spinal segments affected in spinal anesthesia using hyperbaric solutions, an important one being pregnancy. The aforementioned dose should be halved for parturient patients. Other factors include a large volume of anesthetic solution, increases in intra-abdominal pressure, head-down tilt of the patient, coughing or straining by the patient during or immediately following injection, injection at higher segmental levels, a rapid rate of injection, and barbotage (a technique in which cerebrospinal fluid is repeatedly drawn into the syringe during the course of injection to promote mixing).

The most common immediate complication seen following spinal anesthesia is a drop in blood pressure without increase in heart rate. Hypotension is usually mild in young adults but can be severe in parturients and geriatric patients. The cause of hypotension is loss of sympathetic tone. It can be corrected by expanding the circulatory volume with lactated Ringer's solution and administering ephedrine in increments of 5 mg intravenously when necessary (see "Obstetric Patients" in Chap. 19). Profound hypotension and bradycardia together with loss of consciousness and apnea are signs of total spinal anesthesia. In addition to circulatory support, tracheal intubation and controlled ventilation with 100% oxygen are indicated. Recovery should be complete if action is taken promptly.

Sudden and unexpected cardiac arrest during spinal anesthesia has been reported recently, always in patients who have received sedation to supplement an otherwise uneventful spinal anesthetic. It is postulated that loss of sensory input following the onset of spinal anesthesia increases the sensitivity of these patients to sedatives. Unrecognized progressive hypoventilation and hypoxemia may have been the cause of these arrests.

Spinal headache, occasionally accompanied by auditory and

visual disturbances, is an unpleasant side effect of dural puncture. It is due to intracranial hypotension from leakage of cerebrospinal fluid. The incidence of headache is highest in women and least in geriatric patients, and it decreases with the size of the spinal needle used. Treatment should be directed at keeping the patient resting flat in bed, relieving headache with analgesics, and hydrating the patient with liberal fluid intake. If headache is protracted, injection of 10–15 ml of autologous blood into the epidural space at the level of the original lumbar puncture is curative. This procedure, known as *autologous blood patch,* has become an alternative to conservative therapy.

Focal neurologic deficits following spinal anesthesia are reported occasionally. Fortunately they are both minor and transient. The most dreaded, though rare, complication is adhesive arachnoiditis, characterized by nonspecific inflammation of meninges and the spinal cord. The end result is paraplegia. There is no known treatment, only supportive care.

Spinal and epidural hematoma also are rare complications. They usually follow repeated traumatic attempts at lumbar puncture. Bacterial meningitis as a result of poor aseptic technique has also been reported. These complications are preventable.

LUMBAR EPIDURAL ANESTHESIA

The epidural space is a potential space outside the spinal dural sac. It extends from the foramen magnum to the sacrococcygeal membrane and is bounded by the posterior longitudinal ligament anteriorly, the ligamentum flavum posteriorly, and the vertebral laminae, vertebral pedicles, and intervertebral foramina laterally (Fig. 17–4). Local anesthetics deposited into this space can block neural transmission by diffusing intrathecally, by anesthetizing spinal nerve roots, and by blocking spinal nerves as they emerge from the intervertebral foramina.

Epidural anesthesia is suitable for intra-abdominal operations and for those on the perineum and the lower extremities. The most popular approach to the epidural space is the lumbar route using a 16- or 18-gauge Tuohy needle.

For epidural anesthesia, careful placement of the needle is essential. The epidural space can be located by the following method:

1. Position the patient in the lateral decubitus position with the spine well flexed.
2. Raise a skin wheal at an interspace between L2 and S1.
3. Advance the Tuohy needle (Fig. 17–5) with its stylet in place, as described for dural puncture.

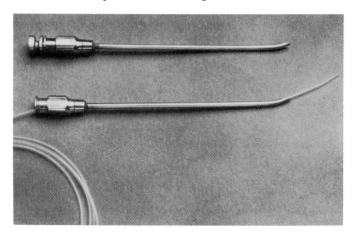

FIGURE 17–5. Tuohy needles. The needle at the bottom has a plastic catheter threaded through its lumen.

4. When the needle is firmly planted in the interspinous ligament, remove the stylet and attach a 5-ml glass syringe half filled with air to the hub of the needle.

5. Advance the needle slowly with one hand while applying gentle pressure to the plunger of the syringe with the other. Note the loss of resistance as the needle enters the epidural space. (When the tip of the needle is in the interspinous ligament or the ligamentum flavum, there is resistance to both advancement of the needle and depression of the plunger. As the needle pierces the ligamentum flavum to enter the epidural space, resistance to both disappears and a click may be felt by the operator. A gush of cerebrospinal fluid after the syringe is detached suggests that the needle has entered the subarachnoid space. Appearance of pure blood, on the other hand, indicates that the needle has entered an epidural vein. In either case the needle should be withdrawn and the attempt repeated at another space.)

Accidental dural puncture can occur without leakage of cerebrospinal fluid through the needle. In order to rule out this complication, a 2- to 3-ml test dose of local anesthetic solution should be injected before the full dose is given. If dural puncture has occurred, onset of spinal anesthesia is usually obvious within 1–2 minutes.

The full dose of lidocaine varies according to the level of anesthesia required and the age of the patient. It is approximately 1.5 ml of 2% lidocaine per spinal segment for a patient of 20 years, 1.25 ml per segment at age 40, 1 ml per segment at age 60, and 0.75 ml per segment at age 80. After injection of the full dose, the needle should be withdrawn and the patient turned to lie supine. The onset of anesthesia is usually rapid, but maximum effect is not seen for 10–15 minutes. Unlike spinal anesthesia, the spread of local anesthetic solution in the epidural space is relatively independent of the force of gravity, the position of the patient, or the mode of injection; however the dose of anesthetic solution should be reduced by one third in paturients, owing to engorgement of epidural veins (see "Obstetric Patients" in Chap. 19). For better control of dose and for continuous epidural anesthesia, a thin catheter can be threaded for 2–3 cm into the lumbar epidural space via the Tuohy needle (Fig. 17–5). Once the catheter is in place, the needle is withdrawn, and repeated doses of lidocaine can be given via the catheter when necessary.

In epidural as well as spinal anesthesia, arterial hypotension is a potential complication and should be managed accordingly. Owing to the large size of the epidural needle, transient backache is also a common complaint. Systemic toxicity, inadvertent dural puncture followed by headache, accidental total spinal, and epidural hematoma are relatively rare complications.

Neither spinal nor epidural anesthesia is effective in alleviating ischemic pain associated with arterial torniquet used on extremities during surgery. Pain can be excruciating, but supplementation of the spinal or epidural anesthesia with intrathecal or epidural opioids can ameliorate this problem.

TREATMENT OF SYSTEMIC TOXICITY

Systemic toxicity is caused by a high blood level of local anesthetic agent caused by administration of a toxic dose, rapid absorption of a nontoxic dose, or accidental intravascular injection. Subtle signs of systemic toxicity include feelings of euphoria, apprehension, restlessness, nausea and vomiting, sensations of heat or cold, and tremor. Signs of frank toxicity are convulsion, postictal coma, respiratory arrest, and circulatory collapse. Most toxic reactions are preventable by keeping the dose within the nontoxic range. If nearly toxic doses are required, addition of epinephrine is indicated. It should be pointed out that systemic effects of epinephrine (pallor, sweating, tachycardia) may mimic the toxic effects of the local anesthetic agent.

Diazepam, given as a preoperative sedative, can increase the convulsion threshold of local anesthetics. It is also the drug of choice in the treatment of central nervous system toxicity. A dose of 5 mg should be given intravenously and repeated as required. Thiopental is also effective in treating convulsion. Since it is not a specific anticonvulsant, an anesthetic dose may be required.

Hypoxemia is always a complication of generalized convulsion because not only does the oxygen requirement of skeletal muscle rise sharply but ventilatory exchange also becomes inadequate as a result of the convulsive activity. If hypoxemia cannot be corrected by administration of oxygen alone, the trachea should be intubated and ventilation should be controlled. Succinylcholine should be used to facilitate tracheal intubation. By inducing muscle paralysis, it also returns oxygen consumption toward normal. It is a very useful agent in the event of such an emergency.

Circulatory collapse may be due to vasomotor paralysis following a massive overdose or to the vasodilating and myocardial depressant effects of local anesthetic agents. It is a grave complication. In addition to controlled ventilation the patient will require expansion of intravascular volume, and possibly myocardial support (e.g., dopamine, 5–50 μg/kg/min).

Care of the Patient During Recovery

Responsibility of the anesthesiologist to his patient extends beyond the phase of emergence, as in most cases the patient is not fully conscious on leaving the operating room. Many of the intraoperative complications, anesthetic as well as surgical, can occur during the early postoperative period. Before being returned to the ward, the patient should be admitted to a post-anesthesia recovery area for close monitoring and care by an experienced nursing staff. Discharge to the ward should be delayed until recovery from the effects of anesthesia is complete and complications are ruled out.

TRANSPORTING THE ANESTHETIZED PATIENT

The means for monitoring and resuscitation are not readily available en route between the operating room and recovery area. Therefore the decision to transfer the patient should not be made unless it is absolutely certain that

1. A patent airway can be maintained.
2. Ventilation is adequate.
3. Cardiovascular function is stable.

During transfer the patient should be positioned in the lateral decubitus position on the stretcher, and the anesthesiologist should be in attendance to look after the airway. If there is any doubt about the adequacy of ventilation, the problem should be corrected before the patient leaves the operating room. Alternatively an endotracheal tube should be left in place so that ventilation can be controlled. Portable oxygen equipment to enrich the inspired atmosphere, pulse oximeter to check oxygenation, and an electrocardiograph equipped with defibrillator to monitor cardiac rhythm should be employed during transport of gravely ill patients.

ARRIVAL IN THE RECOVERY ROOM

Upon arrival in the recovery room, responsibility for the patient's care should be transferred formally to a recovery room nurse. During this transfer the anesthesiologist should supply information essential to proper nursing care as follows:

1. Identify the patient to the nurse.
2. Give a brief summary of the patient's medical history and indicate the nature of the operation.
3. Give a brief summary of the anesthetic technique, the course of the operation, the patient's intake and output in the operating room, and the condition at the end of the operation.
4. Leave instructions on monitoring and laboratory investigation.
5. Leave instructions on the management of pain, fluid therapy, oxygen therapy, and settings of the ventilator if one is in use.

To complete the transfer, the nurse should check the patient's vital signs and state of consciousness and report these to the anesthesiologist. Unless it is contraindicated, the patient should be left lying on one side until fully conscious.

MANAGEMENT OF COMMON POSTANESTHETIC PROBLEMS

Airway Obstruction

During recovery the tongue lying against the posterior pharyngeal wall is the most common cause of upper airway obstruction in the supine unconscious patient. This problem will correct itself if the patient is turned onto one side. Occasionally it is necessary to support the jaw or insert a pharyngeal airway.

Laryngospasm, a less common cause of airway obstruction during this period, is almost always due to irritation of the pharynx or larynx during the "twilight zone" of emergence and recovery (e.g., by the presence of a pharyngeal airway, secretion, debris, or blood). The condition is self-limiting, provided the irritant is removed.

Airway obstruction, from whatever cause, is always an emergency because the end result is hypoventilation and hypoxemia. The precipitating cause must be treated, and the patient should be given oxygen by face mask. If the problem is not readily corrected, tracheal intubation should be considered.

Hypoventilation

Splinting of painful abdominal or chest wounds, narcotic analgesics given for pain, residual neuromuscular paralysis, and airway obstruction are some of the more common causes of hypoventilation seen in the recovery room. The patient who is hypoventilating should be given ventilatory assistance immediately, and airway obstruction should be corrected, as described above. Although appropriate treatment of pain prevents hypoventilation due to splinting, an excessive dose of narcotic analgesic can cause unacceptable respiratory depression, particularly in a patient who has not yet fully recovered from the anesthetic. Naloxone given intravenously is the drug of choice in this last instance. By giving naloxone in increments of 50 μg, an endpoint at which the patient is breathing adequately and yet is pain free can be established.

Perhaps the most common cause of hypoventilation seen in the recovery room in modern anesthetic practice is residual neuromuscular blockade. When a nondepolarizing muscle relaxant is the cause of residual paralysis, an additional dose of anticholinesterase together with a vagolytic agent (e.g., neostigmine and atropine) is indicated. If improvement is not forthcoming the patient should be re-intubated and his ventilation should be controlled. When residual paralysis is due to Phase II succinylcholine block, the problem is pharmacologically more complicated. Although an anticholinesterase like neostigmine will antagonize the Phase II block, it will also enhance any residual Phase I block. Therefore it is simpler to ventilate the lungs mechanically until the neuromuscular junction has regained sensitivity to acetylcholine. In the patient with atypical plasma cholinesterase, the problem is prolonged apnea; in this case ventilation should be controlled until recovery is complete.

Hypoxemia

Cyanosis is a late sign of hypoxemia, of which hypoventilation, airway obstruction, ventilation-perfusion abnormalities, pulmonary edema, and aspiration of gastric contents are some of the causes. The cyanotic patient should be given oxygen by face mask; assisted ventilation should be instituted if indicated. (Management of airway obstruction and hypoventilation is discussed earlier in this chapter, and management of aspiration of gastric contents, in Chap. 16.) Hypoxemia due to ventilation-perfusion inequalities can be successfully treated with an increase in inspired oxygen concentration (see Chap. 10), but arterial desaturation due to pulmonary edema requires treatment of the underlying cause. When pulmonary congestion is the result of fluid overload, treatment with a diuretic is indicated. When congestive heart failure is the cause of poor oxygenation, myocardial support using an inotropic agent is necessary.

Hypotension

The same factors that cause hypotension during surgery can cause hypotension in the recovery phase (see "Hypotension" in Chap. 16). Although hypovolemia is without a doubt the most common cause of hypotension, narcotic analgesics given for pain are a precipitating factor to be considered in the recovery room. All hypotensive patients should receive oxygen supplement, and specific attention should be directed to elimination of the underlying cause.

Hypertension

Arterial hypertension is a not infrequent problem seen in the recovery room. It is particularly common in patients with hypertensive heart disease and systemic atherosclerosis. The more common precipitating factors are pain, distension of urinary bladder, hypoxemia, hypercapnia, and fluid overload. The more serious consequences of uncontrolled hypertension are intracerebral hemorrhage and myocardial ischemia. Obviously treatment should be directed at elimination of the precipitating cause. In the event of a crisis, intravenous administration of an antihypertensive agent is indicated (e.g., diazoxide, 300 mg, intravenously; hydralazine, 10–40 mg, intramuscularly or slowly intravenously; sodium nitroprusside or nitroglycerin infusion by titration).

Shivering

Shivering—ranging from fine muscle tremors to frank convulsion-like clonic contractions—is a common problem during the recovery phase with many anesthetic techniques. The incidence of shivering following halothane anesthesia has been reported to be as high as 50%. Following induction of anesthesia, there is dilation of cutaneous vessels and a fall in the core body temperature. However shivering is only partly explained by this phenomenon. A second contributing factor is loss of cortical inhibition of spinal reflexes during recovery.

Shivering produces a large increase in oxygen demand, which can be met only by similar increases in alveolar ventilation and cardiac output. Since the respiratory and circulatory depressant effects of anesthetic agents last well into the postoperative period, patients recovering from anesthesia may not be able to cope with these demands and may succumb to hypoxemia. Therefore the patient who is shivering should receive oxygen by face mask. Keeping the patient warm could reduce the severity of shivering, and meperidine, 25 mg, given intravenously can abort an attack precipitated by abrupt arousal as a result of pain. Methylphenidate, 10–20 mg intravenously, is also effective, but this agent should not be given to patients in pain. (Methylphenidate is an analeptic without metabolic effects.)

Somnolence

Although somnolence is mostly due to the residual effect of anesthetic agents and to idiosyncrasy, many pre-existing disorders can cause delay in regaining consciousness following general anesthesia—organic disease of the central nervous system (e.g., cerebrovascular accident, head injury, increased intracranial pressure due to space-occupying lesions), acute intoxication due to alcohol or other central nervous system depressants, and disorders of metabolic origin (e.g., myxedema, hepatic encephalopathy, hypoglycemia). Somnolence may also be caused by disorders that develop during the course of the operation. For example, diabetic patients can become hypoglycemic, and hypertensive patients may sustain a cerebrovascular accident. Therefore both organic and anesthetic causes of delay in regaining consciousness should be sought and corrected in all somnolent patients.

Since elimination of inhalation agents via the respiratory tract is slower than normal if alveolar ventilation is inadequate (see "Elimination" in Chap. 3), attention should be directed to keeping the airway clear and maintaining adequate ventilation in somnolent patients. Hyoscine, droperidol, phenothiazines, and benzodiazepines (drugs often included as premedication) can also cause delays in regaining consciousness, particularly in geriatric patients. Usually in these cases it is necessary only to maintain adequate ventilation and allow recovery to occur spontaneously. Physostigmine, 0.5–2 mg given intravenously, can be used to reverse the hypnotic effect of these agents. (Physostigmine is a tertiary amine and the only anticholinesterase that can cross the blood-brain barrier to act on cholinergic sites within the central nervous system.) Narcotic analgesics can also enhance the residual effect of intravenous or inhalation anesthetics to cause somnolence in the recovery phase. If this is the case, careful administration of naloxone can lead to a dramatic arousal.

Delirium

Postoperative delirium is a disconcerting problem. The restless patient can be violent and harm self and attendant. Hypoxemia may not be the most common cause of postoperative delirium, but it is certainly the most dangerous for the patient. It must be ruled out or corrected without delay. Some other causes of postoperative restlessness and excitement are pain, bladder distension, use of ketamine for induction or maintenance, inclusion of hyoscine or phenothiazines in the premedication (particularly in geriatric patients), alcohol or drug withdrawal, and acute intoxication in the unsuspected addict.

As in treatment of other postoperative complications, attention should be directed to eliminating the precipitating cause of delirium. Narcotic analgesics should be given for pain, and the full bladder should be relieved by catheterization. The patient who has received ketamine should be allowed to recover undisturbed in a darkened corner of the recovery room; diazepam, 5–10 mg given intravenously, is the agent of choice for prevention or treatment of unpleasant dreams associated with ketamine. On the other hand, physostigmine, 0.5–2 mg given intravenously, is more effective in the treatment of delirium associated with hyoscine or phenothiazines. Restlessness and excitement due to acute alcohol or drug withdrawal or to acute intoxication may be extremely difficult to diagnose and treat. A trial of methadone can prove successful with the heroin addict, and large doses of diazepam may be necessary to subdue the patient who is intoxicated with LSD or other hallucinogens.

Nausea and Vomiting

Next to pain, nausea and vomiting is the most common complaint in the postoperative period. Although it is a well-known side-effect of narcotic analgesics used in treating pain, other factors are known to be associated with increased incidence and severity of this problem: intra-abdominal or ophthalmic operations, operations on the upper airway during which blood is swallowed, gastric distension from insufflation of air during vigorous positive-pressure ventilation via a face mask, and presence of foreign bodies in the pharynx (e.g., the nasogastric tube). Nausea and vomiting are better prevented than treated. The following points are helpful:

1. Use a pharyngeal pack to minimize the amount of blood swallowed during nose and throat operations.

2. Decompress the stomach by orogastric suction if air has been forced down the esophagus inadvertently.

3. Prescribe an antiemetic to patients undergoing intra-abdominal or ophthalmic operations and to patients known to have had severe nausea and vomiting following anesthesia (e.g., prochlorperazine, 5–10 mg intramuscularly or intravenously).

In the postoperative period prochlorperazine, 5–10 mg, or dimenhydrinate, 25–50 mg, given intramuscularly or intravenously may be used to control troublesome nausea and vomiting; droperidol, 2.5 mg, or metoclopramide, 10 mg, given intravenously are also effective.

MANAGEMENT OF POSTOPERATIVE PAIN

Unrelieved pain can be the cause of many postoperative complications. Splinting of abdominal or chest wounds can lead to hypoventilation, sputum retention, atelectasis, and pneumonia; hypertension and tachycardia in response to pain can be the cause of myocardial ischemia and heart failure; neurohumoral responses to pain can prolong the catabolic phase following surgical trauma and interfere with wound healing. Evidence is emerging that adequate relief of postoperative pain can shorten the hospital stay. With his training and experience, the anesthesiologist should play a leadership role in "acute pain management teams" that are evolving in many institutions.

General Measures

Pain is an inevitable sequela of surgery. Patients differ in their tolerance for pain, and its intensity can vary according to the patient's physical activity. Other than administration of an analgesic, certain general measures can help to reduce the intensity of pain and improve the patient's well-being. They include:

1. Dress wounds on extremities with bulk dressings but avoid restrictive bandages. Restriction of venous return can cause excruciating pain at the site of operation that throbs with each arterial pulsation.

2. Similarly, be sure that plaster casts are not restrictive. Circulation to parts of the extremity distal to the cast should be checked frequently in the immediate postoperative period. Cyanosis and swelling of these parts are signs of restricted venous return; pallor should raise the possibility of arterial obstruction.

3. Support the extremity that has been operated on with pillows so that it is elevated above the patient's heart. Dependency can cause throbbing pain.

4. Instruct the patient who has had an abdominal operation to hug a pillow against the abdomen during coughing and deep breathing exercises but to avoid the use of abdominal splints. By restricting diaphragmatic excursion, these splints can cause basal atelectasis.

5. Treat anxiety with psychological support as well as a tranquilizer if necessary. Unrelieved anxiety can lower pain tolerance.

6. Do not prescribe a hypnotic if sleeplessness is the result of

pain. The semiconscious patient who is still experiencing pain will become delirious.

Oral Analgesics

Acetyl salicylate and acetaminophen are antipyretic analgesics; 650 mg can be given every 4–6 hours for treatment of minor discomfort. Codeine, 15–60 mg, may be added to improve the quality of analgesia. This form of pain relief is suitable only after minor surgery and in later stages after major surgery.

Intramuscular Opiods

Intramuscular injection of meperidine, 1–2 mg/kg, or morphine, 0.1–0.2 mg/kg, every 3–4 hours when necessary, remains the mainstay of the treatment of postoperative pain. This form of pain relief has several limitations:

1. Dose requirement varies widely among patients and in any given patient, depending on physical activity.
2. The therapeutic ratio between an effective analgesic dose and one that causes respiratory depression is relatively narrow. Under the residual effects of anesthesia, patients in the recovery room can be extremely sensitive to the depressant effects of these narcotic analgesics.
3. There is always a significant delay between the time a patient asks for the injection and the time it is given.

In order to improve on the safety of intramuscular opioids, agonist-antagonists with a ceiling effect on respiratory depression have been introduced (e.g., pentazocine, butorphanol, nalbuphine, buprenorphine), but these agents also have limited analgesic potency.

Intravenous Opioids

The quality of analgesia following intravenous opioids is far superior to that after intramuscular injection. Unfortunately this method of pain relief requires close nursing supervision and is practical only in the recovery room or intensive care unit. Meperidine, 10–20 mg, or morphine, 1–2 mg, may be given every 10–20 minutes when necessary.

Patient-controlled analgesia is a more refined method of giving intravenous opioids. Two steps are required for best results.

1. Give incremental doses of morphine or meperidine intravenously until satisfactory analgesia is obtained.
2. Instruct the patient to operate an automated instrument that will dispense 0.5–1 mg of morphine or an equivalent dose of

meperidine intravenously every 5–10 minutes on demand. (In order to prevent overdose, all patient-controlled analgesia devices automatically limit the number of doses a patient can dispense within a given interval. This limit is set by the physician, according to the patient's need.)

This way the patient has total control of his analgesia requirement, which may vary with activity. Experience has shown that the abuse potential of this technique is negligible.

Intrathecal or Epidural Opioids

Morphine, 0.25–0.5 mg deposited in the subarachnoid space, provides analgesia of excellent quality that lasts for 12 hours or more. But repeated dural puncture cannot be justified in long-term care; epidural morphine via an indwelling epidural catheter is more practical. The analgesic effect of morphine, 2–10 mg injected into the lumbar epidural space, can spread to include thoracic dermatomes and has a duration of action of up to 12 hours. Although motor and sympathetic functions are spared, urinary retention is not uncommon. Generalized itching is another annoyance that can be eliminated with a small dose of naloxone. Respiratory depression (delayed for 3–6 hours after intrathecal morphine and for up to 12 hours after epidural morphine) is the most serious complication of these techniques. Therefore supervision of the patient in an acute or subacute care area for the duration is recommended.

Delayed respiratory depression following epidural injection of morphine is due to diffusion of this relatively water-soluble drug into cerebral spinal fluid followed by rostrad spread to act on the respiratory center. Being more lipophilic, fentanyl diffuses into cerebrospinal fluid to a much lesser extent, and delayed respiratory depression is not a problem. Analgesic action following 100 µg of epidural fentanyl lasts only 2–3 hours. Therefore an epidural infusion of 0.5–1 µg/kg/hr is necessary for continuous analgesia.

Epidural Neural Blockade

Continuous infusion of marcaine, 0.25% at 5–8 ml/hr, into the epidural space predates epidural opioids as a method of postoperative pain relief. Some degree of motor and sympathetic blockade is always present; therefore ambulation of the patient is difficult, and hemodynamic instability is a problem. In order to minimize motor and sympathetic blockade, more dilute solutions (e.g., 0.125% marcaine) have been tried with varying success. Some authors have recommended combinations of low-dose marcaine and meperidine or fentanyl as an alternative. This mixed technique is unnecessarily complicated.

Other Modalities

Both infiltration of the wound and simple nerve blocks with marcaine can contribute to pain relief for several hours. By reducing opioid requirement, these techniques can lower the risk of serious respiratory depression. Other procedures that are potentially useful include transcutaneous electrical nerve stimulation (TENS) and instillation of marcaine into the pleural space for pain relief in thoracic and upper abdominal surgery. Results to date have shown that these procedures are only partially effective. New routes for administering opioids are another area under intense investigation. Fentanyl applied to the skin as specially prepared strips is absorbed transdermally and can be used to maintain a sustained analgesic blood level after a latent period of 6–8 hours. Sublingual and transnasal routes are other alternatives.

CARE OF PATIENTS RECOVERING FROM REGIONAL ANESTHESIA

The patient who has received regional anesthesia is free from the problems of general anesthesia and also from pain well into the postoperative period. However, other problems may be encountered.

1. Many patients have been given sedatives from which they must recover.

2. Hypotension accentuated by sudden postural changes is a known complication of spinal or epidural anesthesia.

3. Delays in recovery of motor and sensory functions following nerve blocks and spinal or epidural anesthesia are serious and require immediate attention.

4. Patients still under the effects of regional anesthesia may injure parts of the body without feeling pain (e.g., cigarette burns to fingers that are still numb from brachial plexus block).

Therefore patients should be admitted to the recovery area for observation and protection after regional anesthesia as well. Following major nerve blocks in the upper extremity, the arm and forearm should be protected in a sling. Following major nerve blocks to the lower extremity, the leg should be allowed to rest comfortably on a pillow. In order to avoid postural hypotension due to extensive sympathetic blockade, the patient who has had spinal or epidural anesthesia should be nursed supine (unless that patient is pregnant or has a large intra-abdominal tumor). The supine position minimizes leakage of cerebrospinal fluid following dural puncture and decreases the incidence of "spinal headache." In general, patients who have had regional anesthesia should not be discharged from the recovery room until both motor and sensory functions have been regained.

FITNESS FOR DISCHARGE FROM RECOVERY ROOM

During the patient's stay in the recovery room, an objective method should be used to assess the patient's physical and mental status and progress in recovery. The most popular method is that proposed by J. A. Aldrete and D. Kroulik. In this system the recovery room nurse assigns a score of 0, 1, or 2 for each of five objective signs: activity, respiration, circulation, level of consciousness, and color (Table 18–1). The number of points scored by the patient is recorded every 15 minutes during the first hour of recovery room stay and at longer intervals subsequently if vital signs are stable. Usually discharge from the recovery room should be delayed until the patient has obtained a full score of 10. At the

TABLE 18–1.   POSTANESTHETIC RECOVERY SCORE*

SIGN	CRITERIA	SCORE
Activity	Able to move 4 extremities voluntarily or on command	2
	Able to move 2 extremities voluntarily or on command	1
	Able to move 0 extremities voluntarily or on command	0
Respiration	Able to deep-breathe and cough freely	2
	Dyspneic or with limited breathing	1
	Apneic	0
Circulation	Blood pressure ±20% of preanesthetic level	2
	Blood pressure ±20–50% of preanesthetic level	1
	Blood pressure ±50% of preanesthetic level	0
Consciousness	Fully awake	2
	Arousable on calling	1
	Not responding	0
Color	Pink	2
	Pale, dusky, blotchy, jaundiced, other	1
	Cyanotic	0

* Aldrete JA, Kroulik D: A postanesthetic recovery score. Anesth Analg (Cleve), 49:924, 1970.

end of the stay, the anesthesiologist in charge or his deputy should make a final postoperative visit to assess the patient's condition. Like admission, discharge from the recovery room should be formalized. The anesthesiologist should sign a discharge order after he is satisfied that the patient has recovered fully from the anesthetic.

Anesthetic Management of Obstetric, Pediatric, Geriatric, and Ambulatory Patients

Anesthetic techniques are usually modified according to the nature of the operation and the medical and physiologic condition of the patient. Obstetric, pediatric, geriatric, and ambulatory patients are large subgroups of surgical patients the anesthesiologist meets daily in clinical practice. These patients have unique problems that require special attention. In this chapter, general principles of management in each group are reviewed.

OBSTETRIC PATIENTS

During pregnancy, the mother undergoes certain physiologic changes necessary to cope with demands of the unborn child. Any interference with systemic functions of the mother has an indirect effect on the fetus. Therefore sound anesthesia management of obstetric patients should be based on a clear understanding of maternal and fetal physiology and of related changes in drug sensitivity.

THE MOTHER

Respiratory System

In the pregnant patient near term, oxygen consumption increases by 20% and metabolic rate by 15%. Owing to encroachment of the gravid uterus on the diaphragm, residual volume, expiratory reserve volume, and functional residual capacity (FRC) are decreased by as much as 20%. However, tidal volume is increased by 40%, respiratory rate by 15%, and alveolar ventilation by 65%. This degree of hyperventilation is reflected in a resting $PaCO_2$ of 30–35 mm Hg. Since respiratory alkalosis is compensated by urinary excretion of bicarbonate, arterial pH remains normal.

As a result of this large fall in FRC, impairment of arterial oxygenation following induction of anesthesia is worse in parturients than in nonpregnant patients. Therefore, a higher inspired oxygen concentration should be given during the course of anesthesia. Despite an increase in cardiac output, the increase in alveolar ventilation and fall in FRC mean an increase in the rate of alveolar uptake of inhalation agents. An unexpectedly deep level of anesthesia may occur rapidly in the parturient if a high concentration of volatile agent is administered, particularly if it is an insoluble agent (see "Alveolar Uptake" in Chap. 3).

Circulatory System

During pregnancy there is a steady increase in blood volume. Although circulating volume starts to decline after the eighth lunar month, it is still 25% above nonpregnant values at term. Since increase in plasma volume is larger than that in red cell volume, hematocrit will fall to as low as 35%.

Cardiac output also increases steadily during pregnancy and follows a trend similar to that of blood volume. During labor and with each contraction, cardiac output increases even further, so that it is 45% above normal during the second stage of labor. These changes in cardiac output, however, are modified by postures assumed by the patient. If she is allowed to lie supine, compression of the vena cava by the gravid uterus will obstruct venous return to the heart, reduce cardiac output, and cause maternal hypotension and fetal acidosis. Fetal hypoxemia and acidosis are further aggravated by hypoperfusion of the uteroplacental circulation resulting from partial compression of the aorta by the gravid uterus. This supine hypotension syndrome becomes a problem approximately half way through the pregnancy.

Increase in blood volume is a safeguard against blood loss and allows the parturient to tolerate a 20% loss of circulating volume without transfusion. Supine hypotension, however, is dangerous for both mother and fetus. Both general and spinal or epidural anesthesia can increase the severity of this problem. Fortunately it can be alleviated by manually displacing the uterus to the left or by elevating the right hip of the mother with a wedge.

Gastrointestinal System

As the diaphragm rises with the growing uterus, the gastroesophageal sphincter becomes incompetent and allows reflux of stomach contents into the lower esophagus, particularly when the mother assumes the supine posture. Furthermore both gastric emptying time and gastric acidity are increased during pregnancy. Thus the risk of regurgitation and aspiration of stomach contents is increased during pregnancy, although the stage at which this risk becomes important is unclear. Premedication with 1/3 molar sodium bicitrate and an H_2-receptor antagonist plus rapid-sequence induction are recommended from the second trimester if general anesthesia is contemplated.

Other Functional Changes

The parturient is more sensitive to inhalation anesthetics, and minimum alveolar concentration decreases by as much as 40% during pregnancy. Plasma cholinesterase activity is lower than normal; but clinically important prolonged apnea following administration of succinylcholine is rare. Owing to engorgement of epidural veins, volume of the epidural space is smaller than normal in pregnant patients. Therefore the dose of local anesthetic used for epidural anesthesia should be reduced by one third at term.

THE FETUS

Effects of Anesthetic Drugs

The fetus is totally dependent on the integrity of the uteroplacental circulation for gas exchange. All anesthetic agents, by acting directly or indirectly on this special circulation, can affect the well-being of the fetus. Ultra-short-acting barbiturates can cause a small and transient fall in maternal blood pressure and uterine blood flow. Similarly all volatile agents in high concentrations can cause marked maternal hypotension, uterine hypoperfusion, and fetal hypoxemia. Under a low dose (e.g., 0.5–1% of halothane or equivalent doses of enflurane or isoflurane), however, normal uterine blood flow and normal fetal respiration are maintained despite a mild fall in maternal blood pressure. Local anesthetics, on the other hand, have no direct effects on the uteroplacental circulation, but the profound sympathetic blockade produced when these agents are injected into the intrathecal or epidural space can aggravate the severity of the supine hypotension syndrome and cause fetal acidosis.

Not only can anesthetic drugs cause fetal hypoxemia, but also maternal anxiety or stress, by stimulating the release of catechol-amine, can lead to vasoconstriction of the uteroplacental circulation and fetal asphyxia. Similarly, hyperventilation by mechanical means can produce reduction in uterine blood flow.

Most anesthetic drugs can cross the placental barrier. In addition to their indirect effect on fetal respiration discussed above, they have direct effects on the neonate that can threaten survival. The effects of the commonly used agents are listed below:

1. All *barbiturates* cross the placental barrier readily, and high doses of these agents given to the mother during labor have been associated with neonatal respiratory depression, lethargy, and failure to feed. For this reason, the induction dose of thiopental should be limited to 4 mg/kg in the parturient patient. Similarly high doses of *diazepam* given to the mother can cause neonatal flaccidity and hypothermia, and high doses of *ketamine* can cause neonatal depression. Nevertheless doses up to 10 mg of diazepam and 1 mg/kg of ketamine are considered safe.

2. Anesthetic concentrations of *inhalation agents* can lead to neonatal depression by two mechanisms: causing maternal hypotension and uterine hypoperfusion and crossing the placental barrier to act directly on the central nervous system of the fetus. Analgesic concentrations administered for short durations, on the other hand, are free of any depressant effects on the newborn.

3. All long-acting *narcotic analgesics* can cause neonatal respiratory depression and apnea when they are given to the mother within 4 hours of delivery. Although this depressant action of meperidine, the most popular narcotic analgesic in obstetrics, is not obvious for at least 1 hour after intramuscular injection, this effect is immediate after intravenous injection.

4. *Muscle relaxants* are highly ionized at physiologic pH. With the exception of gallamine, they do not cross the placental barrier readily. Neonatal muscle weakness has not been reported after clinical doses of these agents.

5. Among *local anesthetics* lidocaine or mepivacaine given for epidural anesthesia during delivery (but not bupivacaine, chloroprocaine, or etidocaine) has the potential to cause transient and minor neurobehavioral abnormalities in the neonate. However all these agents have been used safely in obstetric practice without any permanent sequelae on newborn infants.

6. The aforementioned effects of anesthetic drugs on the fetus at term have been well documented, but their effects on organogenesis in the fetus during early pregnancy are unclear. What is clear though is that the incidence of congenital abnormalities following a single exposure to anesthesia is not increased, but the incidence of spontaneous abortion following operations under general anesthesia in the first or second trimester is.

Fetal Monitoring

In short, anesthetic agents act on both the mother and the fetus. Therefore monitoring the fetus is as important as monitoring the mother during the course of anesthesia. During labor, sampling *fetal scalp capillary blood for pH* determination is the most accurate method of assessing fetal well-being. A pH greater than 7.25 is normal, while one less than 7.20 means fetal acidosis; however, this method of assessment is invasive. Checking fetal heart rate in relation to uterine contraction remains the mainstay of fetal monitoring. This can be done intermittently with a stethoscope or continuously with electronic devices.

Normal fetal heart rate is between 120 and 160 beats/min. It slows with uterine contraction and increases with uterine relaxation. The *early deceleration* pattern, in which slowing begins and ends simultaneously with contraction, is due to compression of the fetal head and is normal. The *late deceleration* pattern, in which slowing beings late in contraction and ends after contraction has subsided, is abnormal and indicates fetal hypoxemia. In *variable deceleration*, slowing is totally out of phase with contraction; this pattern is thought to be due to umbilical cord compression. It is associated with fetal compromise if (1) it lasts more than 60 seconds, (2) the fetal heart rate is below 60 beats/min at the nadir, or (3) the fetal heart rate is 60 beats below the baseline value. In addition to the stress patterns discussed, *absence of variability* in baseline rate is also an ominous sign.

REGIONAL ANESTHESIA

Regional anesthesia is suitable both for analgesia in the first stage of labor and for delivery. The most popular technique in use today is lumbar epidural anesthesia. When this technique is used for pain relief, it should be administered only when labor is well-established in the active phase. An epidural catheter is usually left in place so that additional doses can be given intermittently as required or continuously (see "Lumbar Epidural Anesthesia" in Chap. 17).

Early in the first stage of labor, pain is caused by uterine contractions and cervical dilation. During this stage pain impulses travel centrally with sympathetic fibers of spinal nerves arising from T10–12. Only 8–10 ml of 0.25% bupivacaine (or equianalgesic doses of other agents) given at the lumbar level is required to provide adequate analgesia at this stage. Late in the first stage and during delivery, additional discomfort is caused by distension of the birth canal and perineum. These structures are innervated by somatic fibers arising from S2–S4. Approximately 12–14 ml of bupivacaine given at the lumbar level is required to provide both analgesia and relaxation for delivery. When lumbar epidural anesthesia is employed for cesarean section, approximately 20 ml of anesthetic solution is necessary for relaxation of the abdominal musculature.

A major complication of epidural anesthesia in obstetrics is aggravation of the supine hypotension syndrome by sympathetic blockade. Severity of hypotension can be minimized by administering a fluid load (give 1000 ml of lactated Ringer's solution before the onset of blockade), by injecting the local anesthetic solution with the mother lying on her side, and by placing a wedge under the mother's right hip after she is turned supine. If necessary, ephedrine, 5 mg, can be given intravenously in increments to maintain normotension.

Spinal anesthesia is also popular in obstetrics. Usually 5 mg of hyperbaric tetracaine or 30 mg of hyperbaric lidocaine is given for vaginal delivery only. Unfortunately the incidence of spinal headache is considerable, despite the use of small-gauge spinal needles.

GENERAL ANESTHESIA

General anesthesia is becoming less popular for delivery or cesarean section in recent years, but there is no convincing evidence that it has adverse effects on the acid-base status of newborn infants. Although infants born under general anesthesia have lower neurobehavioral scores than those born under regional anesthesia, this difference disappears by 24 hours. Nevertheless, for reasons discussed earlier, the following modifications in technique are recommended:

1. Owing to the high incidence of gastric reflux, obstetric patients should be premedicated with 1/3 molar sodium bicitrate and an H_2-receptor antagonist. Rapid-sequence induction is the method of choice.

2. The dose of thiopental should be limited to 4 mg/kg. In order to minimize fetal uptake of thiopental, it should be given at the beginning of a uterine contraction, when uteroplacental blood flow is least.

3. As an alternative to thiopental, some anesthesiologists prefer to use ketamine, 1 mg/kg, for induction; but there is not enough evidence to favor one or the other.

4. A mixutre of 50% oxygen in nitrous oxide and 0.5% halothane (or equivalent doses of enflurane or isoflurane) should be used to

maintain anesthesia. The use of narcotic analgesics should be avoided until the fetus is delivered and the cord clamped.

5. Hyperventilation should be avoided. Hypocapnia and the mechanical effect of positive-pressure ventilation can decrease uteroplacental blood flow.

6. A wedge should be placed under the patient's right hip, or the surgeon should displace the uterus manually to the left. These maneuvers will reduce the incidence and severity of the supine hypotension syndrome.

PEDIATRIC PATIENTS

Children are not small adults. They are distinguishable by certain anatomic, physiologic, and psychological characteristics that demand special consideration throughout the course of anesthesia, from preparation to recovery.

Preparation for Anesthesia

In order to minimize psychic trauma caused by separation of parents and child, many minor pediatric procedures are done on an outpatient basis. Selection criteria for outpatients are similar in children and adults, but not in infants born prematurely (see "Ambulatory Patients," below). Infants in this group are prone to develop sleep apnea in the postoperative period. They should not be selected for outpatient surgery until they have caught up with their peers in growth and development.

Regardless of whether the child is an inpatient or an outpatient, careful assessment, as outlined in Chapter 12, should be carried out. During the interview, willingness to listen and to alleviate the child's fears is the best way to gain his confidence.

Since small children can become dehydrated quickly, it is important to modify the rules of fasting before a scheduled operation. Small infants should be allowed to have 5% glucose by mouth until 4 hours before the operation, and older children, clear fluids until 6 hours before.

Most small children find the hospital environment strange and frightening, and preoperative sedation is advisable. In order to avoid the unpleasantness of an injection, the oral route is preferred (e.g., diazepam elixir, 0.3 mg/kg 30–60 minutes before the operation). Use of atropine to block vagal reflexes is still popular in most pediatric centers, but it can be given intravenously at the time of induction. (The dose of atropine is 0.02 mg/kg but not to exceed 0.6 mg.)

Monitoring

The principle of monitoring is the same whether the patient is an adult or a child (see Chap. 14). However, use of the precordial or esophageal stethoscope is more popular in pediatric patients and provides a means of monitoring both heart sounds and breath sounds continuously. Monitoring body temperature is considered mandatory in children because they are more prone than adults to develop hypothermia. The incidence of malignant hyperthermia is also higher in younger patients; this is another indication for monitoring body temperature.

Induction of Anesthesia

Given the choice, most children under 5 years *would* prefer inhalation to intravenous induction. This technique is described in Chapter 15, but some modifications are necessary:

1. Most children find the procedure more acceptable if they are given a full explanation and are shown the components of the anesthetic circuit. Some may express the wish to hold on to the mask themselves.

2. Children may find the smell of volatile agents, even in low concentrations, offensive. They should be given a mixture of 50% nitrous oxide in oxygen first; anesthetic vapor should be added only after the onset of drowsiness.

3. In order to avoid the unpleasantness of the needle, the intravenous infusion can be established after onset of surgical anesthesia.

At times, intravenous induction is more appropriate (e.g., in children who have a previously established intravenous infusion, in those who are willing, and when rapid-sequence induction is indicated). The method has been described in Chapter 15; little modification is necessary. Other alternatives include 20–30 mg/kg of 10% methohexital given rectally or 5–8 mg/kg of ketamine given intramuscularly. The last two techniques are particularly useful for a frightened child who is totally uncooperative.

Tracheal Intubation

Indications for tracheal intubation in pediatric practice are the same as those stated in Chapter 13. Age itself is not a factor in tracheal intubation, but the technique must be modified somewhat for the following reasons:

1. In infants the larynx is high up in the neck between C2 and

C4, the glottis is farther anterior, and the epiglottis is long and tends to overhang the glottis. Direct laryngoscopy with a straight blade is the method of choice in infants under 6 months of age.

2. The larynx of infants and young children is funnel-shaped; the narrowest point being the round cricoid cartilage. Pressure from a snug-fitting tube can cause subglottic edema. Therefore endotracheal tubes used in pediatric practice should be of a size that will pass through the glottis easily, to allow a small air leak when positive pressure is applied to the airway. Usually uncuffed endotracheal tubes are used in infants and children, but a cuffed tube may be used in older children. In order to avoid barotrauma to the trachea, care should be exercised not to overinflate the cuff in the latter instance.

3. In children, the inner diameter of orotracheal tubes can be estimated according to the following formula: (age in years ÷ 4) + 4.5 mm. Since this formula is not infallible, tubes 0.5 mm larger and 0.5 mm smaller than the estimated size should be readily available.

4. Usually tracheal intubation is accomplished in infants and children after induction of anesthesia and administration of succinylcholine. However, in premature infants and neonates tracheal intubation before induction of anesthesia may be the safest method of maintaining a clear airway.

Maintenance of Anesthesia

Jackson-Rees' modification of the Ayre's T-piece is a popular anesthetic circuit in pediatric practice. It is suitable for both spontaneous and controlled ventilation (see "Ayre's T-Piece" in Chap. 8).

When the patient is allowed to breathe spontaneously, anesthesia is maintained with oxygen, nitrous oxide, and a volatile agent such as halothane, enflurane, or isoflurane. When profound muscle relaxation is required, a muscle relaxant is added and ventilation is controlled. The experienced pediatric anesthesiologist may choose to replace the volatile agent with a narcotic analgesic when a muscle relaxant is being used. The agents and dosages commonly used in pediatric anesthesia are shown in Table 19–1.

Accidental development of hypothermia during the course of the operation is a common anesthetic complication in pediatric practice. Thermostatically controlled water mattresses with temperature set at 40° C, solar blankets, and heated baths for intravenous fluids should be employed routinely to minimize this complication. Humidifying and warming the anesthetic fresh gas is another effective measure for maintaining normothermia during lengthy operations.

TABLE 19–1.   ANESTHETIC AGENTS COMMONLY USED IN
PEDIATRICS

AGENTS	DOSE
Intravenous Agents	
Thiopental	5 mg/kg IV
Methohexital	2 mg/kg IV
Ketamine	2 mg/kg IV, 5–8 mg/kg IM
Muscle Relaxants	
Succinylcholine	1 mg/kg IV, 2 mg/kg IM
d-Tubocurarine	
Initial dose	0.2–0.5 mg/kg IV
Subsequent dose	One fifth of initial dose IV
Pancuronium	
Initial dose	0.05–0.1 mg/kg IV
Subsequent dose	One fifth of initial dose IV
Atracurium	
Initial dose	0.3–0.5 mg/kg IV
Subsequent dose	One fifth of initial dose IV
Vecuronium	
Initial dose	0.05–0.1 mg/kg IV
Subsequent dose	One fifth of initial dose IV
Agents for Reversal of Nondepolarizing Block	
Atropine	0.02 mg/kg IV
Neostigmine	0.05 mg/kg IV
Narcotic Analgesics	
Morphine	
To supplement anesthesia	0.01–0.03 mg/kg IV
For postoperative pain	0.05–0.1 mg/kg IM
Meperidine	
To supplement anesthesia	0.2 mg/kg IV
For postoperative pain	1 mg/kg IM
Codeine	
For postoperative pain	1 mg/kg IM (up to 50 mg)
Opiate Antagonist	
Naloxone	0.01 mg/kg

Emergence and Recovery

The emergence of pediatric patients from anesthesia is similar
to that described for other patients, with one exception: the trachea of infants and children should always be extubated only after
the return of the cough and gag reflexes. This prevents the development of laryngospasm and minimizes the risk of aspiration.

In the recovery room, premature infants and neonates should

be nursed in a heated incubator supplied with humidified oxygen-enriched air, and older children should receive oxygen by face mask. A narcotic analgesic administered before the child is fully roused is indicated, particularly if none has been given during the operation.

Postintubation subglottic edema, characterized by tachypnea, tachycardia, a croupy cough, and signs of upper airway obstruction, is a potential complication in young children following endotracheal anesthesia. The onset may be immediate or delayed. Nursing the patient in a croupette supplied with a cool, humidified, and oxygen-rich atmosphere may be the only treatment required when edema of the airway is mild. Administration of racemic epinephrine by aerosol, with or without dexamethasone, 4–8 mg intravenously, is indicated in more severe cases. (The dose of racemic epinephrine is 0.25–0.50 ml of a 2.25% solution in 3 ml of normal saline.) If improvement is not forthcoming, re-intubation should be considered. Edema subsides with time, and extubation is usually successful in 36–72 hours. On rare occasions, tracheostomy is necessary to relieve persistent and progressive airway obstruction.

GERIATRIC PATIENTS

With high standards of living, improved public health measures, and better personal hygiene, life expectancy in North America and Western Europe has increased from 60+ years to 70+. As a result many of the resources in health sciences research have been devoted to unlocking the secret of aging. This last decade has also seen the birth of geriatric medicine, a new discipline specializing in providing health care for elderly persons.

Although geriatric patients have reduced reserves in all organic functions, old age is not a disease. Elderly persons are frequently victims of degenerative or neoplastic disease; those living alone are prone to be malnourished; and many are taking a large number of drugs. But there is no disease process that strikes elderly patients alone. The principles of anesthesia practice are the same regardless of age, but some problems are unique to this age group:

1. The superficial veins of many elderly patients have poor connective tissue support and are fragile. It may be difficult to maintain an intravenous infusion for prolonged periods. Occasionally cannulation of a central vein is the only recourse.

2. Many elderly patients are edentulous and have sunken cheeks. To find a form-fitting face mask for these patients is sometimes difficult. It may be impossible to administer an inhalation anesthetic except via endotracheal intubation.

3. Elderly patients are more prone to have ischemic heart disease, and all of them have some degree of systolic hypertension. In the absence of surgical stimulation, blood pressure in the anesthetized geriatric patient tends to be low, but surgical stimulation in light planes of anesthesia can cause a steep rise in blood pressure. Therefore careful adjustment of the depth of anesthesia according to need is imperative.

4. Closing capacity as well as alveolar-arterial oxygen tension difference increases with age. The elderly patient should be given a higher inspired oxygen concentration to maintain normal arterial oxygenation under anesthesia.

5. Elderly patients have a marked reduction in muscle mass. They are sensitive not only to the effects of muscle relaxants but also to drugs that rely on redistribution to muscle for termination of action. Futhermore, hepatic blood flow, hepatobiliary function, renal plasma flow, glomerular filtration, and renal tubular function are depressed in elderly persons, so drug metabolism and elimination are impaired. During the course of anesthesia, drugs should be given slowly and in small increments so that dose can be titrated against effect.

6. Many elderly persons medicate themselves with an unnecessarily large number of drugs, and drug toxicity is a common occurrence in this group. These problems must be carefully assessed so that abnormalities can be corrected in the preoperative period.

7. Hospitalization can cause severe disorientation, and general anesthesia can precipitate an acute attack of psychosis in senile patients. Although the avoidance of drugs such as hyoscine and droperidol in elderly patients has reduced the incidence of these problems, frequent visits by close relatives should also be encouraged. Since the use of central nervous system depressants can be avoided altogether with regional anesthesia, these techniques should be considered when they are applicable.

8. Elderly patients who are bedridden are predisposed to respiratory infection and deep vein thrombosis. In the postoperative period, early ambulation and vigorous physiotherapy should be instituted to prevent complications associated with immobility.

There is a smaller margin for error in the anesthetic management of geriatric patients. They should be carefully evaluated and meticulously prepared before anesthesia and surgery. During the course of the anesthetic, vigilance and diligence are required in monitoring depth of anesthesia and the well-being of the patient.

AMBULATORY PATIENTS

Ambulatory care offers the opportunity to treat patients at a reduced cost and without separating them from family. This concept is gaining popularity in the practice of surgery. Most short procedures that do not interfere with the patient's ability to eat or walk can be done in a well-equipped outpatient surgical clinic.

Assessment and Preparation of the Patient

Candidates for outpatient surgery should receive the same intensive preoperative assessment recommended for inpatients. Ideally it should be done by the anesthesiologist, but the patient's surgeon or a family physician who is knowledgeable about selection criteria can act as surrogate. All patients in Class I of the American Society of Anesthesiologists' Classification of Physical Status are acceptable for outpatient surgery, but only medically stable patients in Class II or III whose systemic illness or its treatment is not affected by the anesthetic or the operation are suitable candidates. (For instance, a stable diabetic treated with an oral hypoglycemic agent is suitable but one treated with insulin is not.) The patient's socioeconomic profile is also an important factor in determining suitability. There must be a responsible adult at home to care for the patient, and this guardian must be capable of following instructions.

Anesthetic Considerations

Like inpatients, surgical outpatients should take nothing by mouth the night before the scheduled operation. Premedication is usually omitted.

Local or regional anesthesia is an excellent choice for outpatient surgery. These techniques are associated with no clouding of sensorium, little or no nausea and vomiting, and good pain relief that persists well into the postoperative period. Local infiltrations, peripheral nerve blocks, brachial plexus block, and intravenous regional anesthesia are popular techniques; epidural anesthesia using a short-acting agent (chloroprocaine) may be considered; but spinal anesthesia is contraindicated owing to the high incidence of spinal headache.

If general anesthesia is elected, techniques associated with a short recovery time and minimal residual sedation should be employed. Therefore inhalation induction is superior to intravenous induction, and methohexital or propofol, rather than thiopental, is the agent of choice for intravenous induction. Likewise fentanyl or alfentanil is more suitable than morphine as an analgesic supplement. Outpatient anesthesia is not a contraindication to tracheal intubation and controlled ventilation; however, if succinylcholine is used to facilitate intubation of the trachea, precurarization is recommended to prevent muscle pain.

Postoperative Care

The surgical outpatient should be allowed to recover from the anesthesia just as any other patient is, and discharge from the hospital should be delayed until the patient is fully ambulatory without dizziness and is able to eat a light meal. The patient should

---

University Hospital

INSTRUCTIONS FOR SURGICAL OUTPATIENTS REQUIRING GENERAL OR LOCAL ANAESTHESIA

1. Please report to Patient Registration, Main Floor, University Hospital, on:

   Date . . . . at (Time) . . . .

   IT IS IMPORTANT FOR YOU TO BE PUNCTUAL SO THAT NECESSARY PREPARATIONS CAN BE MADE BEFORE ANAESTHESIA AND SURGERY.

BEFORE COMING TO HOSPITAL:

2. If your health changes or if you develop a cold, flu or any chest disease during the week before your operation, please notify your doctor (surgeon or gynaecologist) before you come to the hospital.

3. **DO NOT** bring large sums of money or unnecessary jewellery with you to the hospital. The hospital cannot assume responsibility for their safekeeping.

4. **YOU MUST ARRANGE FOR A RESPONSIBLE ADULT TO ACCOMPANY YOU HOME** following your operation. You must not drive a motor vehicle. You must go home with your companion by private vehicle or by taxi and **NOT** by public transportation.

5. Please **BRING** the names of all the medicine (liquid, tablets or pills) you are taking or their containers with you so that they can be identified.

6. Please **BRING** your first morning specimen of urine with you. Any clean jar thoroughly washed with soap and water, is a suitable container.

7. **DO NOT EAT OR DRINK ANYTHING FROM MIDNIGHT THE NIGHT BEFORE YOU COME TO THE HOSPITAL.** If you eat or drink after midnight, you may vomit during the anaesthetic and this can be dangerous; it may be necessary to reschedule your surgery.

AFTER YOUR OPERATION:

8. Despite the fact that you may feel fully conscious following an anaesthetic, your judgement and reactions will be impaired. **DO NOT** drive any motorized or mechanical vehicle or perform any task that requires skill, coordination or judgement for at least 24 hours following your anaesthetic.

9. Alcohol, sedatives, tranquilizers and all related drugs will increase the after-effect of your anaesthetic. You are advised **NOT** to drink any alcoholic beverages or take any such drugs for at least 24 hours following your anaesthetic. If in doubt, consult your doctor or anaesthetist.

10. Nausea, sore throat and muscle pain are common the day after an anaesthetic. If you feel there are unusual effects from the anaesthetic or the operation, **CONSULT** your doctor or the Emergency Department of University Hospital.

I, ... have read and understand the above instructions.

Date . . . .
                                        Signature

                                        Address . . . .

THIS FORM IS PART OF THE HOSPITAL CHART AND MUST BE SIGNED BEFORE SURGERY CAN BEGIN

If you are being seen in the Out Patient Department, University Hospital, please give the signed original to clerk or nurse.

If you are being seen by a physician outside University Hospital, please bring signed original with you when you come to University Hospital for your surgery. In either case, retain the copy for your own use.

FIGURE 19–1.   Preoperative and postoperative instructions for the surgical outpatient.

be given a prescription for oral analgesics and should be escorted home by a responsible adult.

Since the residual effect of anesthetic drugs can last 24 hours or more, the ambulatory surgical outpatient should be instructed not to perform any tasks that require quick reflexes or judgment (e.g., operating a motor vehicle or machinery or signing a business contract) for at least 24 hours after recovering from anesthesia. The residual effect of anesthetics produces poor tolerance of central nervous system depressants, so the patient should be instructed not to take any alcoholic beverages or tranquilizers for the next 24 hours. In addition, he should be warned of the common side-effects of general anesthesia (nausea or vomiting, sore throat, muscle pain). The patient should also be given the telephone number of the anesthesiologist or the surgeon and told to report any untoward complications immediately. In order to ensure that there is no misunderstanding, both preoperative and postoperative instructions should be written out for the patient when ambulatory surgery is contemplated (Fig. 19–1).

Fluid and Electrolyte Requirements of Surgical Patients

All surgical patients are required to abstain from oral intake for several hours before and after an operation, and in some cases, for even longer periods. Maintenance of fluid and electrolyte homeostasis with intravenous fluid is therefore critical for these patients' well-being. Not only should basal requirements be met, but pre-existing deficits and ongoing losses should be replaced; that is,

$$\text{Total requirement} = \frac{\text{Basal}}{\text{requirement}} + \frac{\text{Pre-existing}}{\text{deficit}} + \frac{\text{Ongoing}}{\text{losses}}$$

In this chapter a practical approach to fluid and electrolyte therapy is set forth. A discussion on the use of blood and plasma products is reserved for Chapter 21.

BASAL REQUIREMENTS

Water

A healthy adult consumes approximately 2500 ml of water per day, of which 1500 ml is ingested as liquid, 800 ml is part of solid food, and 200 ml is derived from oxidation of carbohydrate and fat. Normal daily losses are 1500 ml as urine and another 1000 ml as insensible loss (800 ml via the skin and respiratory tract and 200 ml in feces). Thus intake and output are in balance. With fluid deprivation, the body can conserve water by increasing urinary concentration of solutes and decreasing urine volume; however, the normal kidney can concentrate urine only to a maximum specific gravity of 1.035. Approximately 500–600 ml of urine is still required to excrete 600 mOsm of solute each day. Although fluid retention is part of the metabolic response to injury, it is normally safe to calculate the basal water requirement of the patient undergoing surgery according to these guidelines:

4 ml/kg/hr for the first 10 kg body weight
2 ml/kg/hr for the second 10 kg body weight
1 ml/kg/hr for each additional kilogram of body weight.

Sodium

The salt intake of a normal person is 50–100 mEq per day. Sodium homeostasis is maintained mainly by excretion in urine; a small amount is lost through skin in sweat and some is lost through the intestine. Under conditions of reduced intake, the kidneys can conserve sodium and excrete urine that is practically free of sodium, but the surgical patient benefits from receiving the normal daily requirement. If all of the basal fluid intake is given as 0.3% saline and 3.3% dextrose in water, the daily requirement of sodium will be met.

Potassium

The ability of the kidneys to conserve potassium is poor. In order to avoid a deficit, a daily basal requirement of 30–60 mEq of potassium must be met. However, during the operation and in the early postoperative phase, tissue catabolism is accompanied by mobilization of a large amount of potassium. Therefore, administration of potassium in the first 2 postoperative days usually is not necessary unless a deficit can be demonstrated. Thereafter, a maintenance dose of 0.5–1 mEq/kg per day should be given intravenously if the patient has not resumed oral feeding.

PRE-EXISTING DEFICITS

Owing to the nature of the surgical illness, many patients present with pre-existing deficits of water and salt. A mild degree of fluid loss produces no symptoms but a 5% loss of body weight in fluid is reflected in poor skin turgor, dry oral mucous membranes, longitudinal furrowing of the tongue, decreased intraocular tension, oliguria, tachycardia, and orthostatic hypotension. Collapsed peripheral veins, sunken eyeballs, cold extremities, frank hypotension, and clouded sensorium are signs of more severe volume depletion. An acute drop in body weight is an accurate reflection of the amount of fluid lost externally. Similarly frequency of vomiting or diarrhea, biochemical changes (see below), and measurement of central venous or pulmonary capillary wedge pressure can be used to estimate the magnitude and character of fluid loss.

Water and Sodium Deficits

Many patients who require surgery have combined water and sodium deficits. For convenience, these deficits can be classified into three categories, according to the amount of sodium in the fluid: (1) loss of isotonic water and sodium, (2) loss of excess water, or (3) loss of excess sodium.

In general, *isotonic losses of water and salt* occur through the gastrointestinal tract, by vomiting, diarrhea, nasogastric suction, and so forth. Other losses include fluids sequestered in the lumen of bowels and at the site of injury (so-called third-space losses). As fluid is lost, contraction of plasma volume leads to hemoconcentration, decreased renal blood flow, prerenal azotemia, metabolic acidosis, hyperkalemia, and eventually, circulatory collapse. Urinary sodium concentration is often less than 10 mEq/L, but serum sodium concentration is normal. Weight lost acutely is the best estimate of the amount of external fluid loss. Otherwise, central venous or pulmonary capillary wedge pressure measurement should be used as a guide to replacement therapy. If plasma sodium concentration is normal, the ideal replacement fluid is a balanced salt solution such as lactated Ringer's solution.

The most common cause of *excess water loss* is inadequate water intake. Dehydration may be aggravated by excessive insensible loss in a hot climate or during febrile illness, and it is frequently observed in patients who are debilitated and living alone. Diuresis due to glycosuria and diabetes insipidus are less common causes of excess water loss; in addition to hypovolemia, affected patients have hypernatremia. Since normal serum sodium concentration is approximately 140 mEq/L, the volume of deficit can be estimated according to the equation

$$\frac{\text{Volume}}{\text{deficit}} = \left(\frac{\text{Measured serum Na conc.}}{140} - 1\right) \times \text{Total body water}$$

(Total body water is approximately 50% of body weight in women and 60% in men.) This volume should be replaced with 5% dextrose. However, in hypotensive patients, a hypotonic saline solution should be used instead (e.g., 0.3% saline in 3.3% dextrose).

Excess sodium loss is characterized by hyponatremia. Surgical causes of excess sodium loss are rare. Hyponatremia is usually the result of replacing isotonic deficits with a hypotonic solution. If serum concentratrion falls below 110 mEq/L, cerebral edema and convulsions (water intoxication) may occur. Normal serum sodium concentration is 140 mEq/L; the amount of deficit can be calculated according to the equation

$$\text{Na deficit} = (140 - \text{Measured serum Na conc.}) \times \text{Total body water}$$

Isotonic saline, which has 154 mEq sodium per liter, is the ideal replacement fluid when hyponatremia is mild. When water intoxication is imminent, 5% saline should be infused slowly until symptoms have abated. Hypertonic saline can cause rapid expansion of intravascular volume, leading to pulmonary congestion. Rapid or prolonged infusion of 5% saline is never indicated.

If volume deficit is a common complication of many surgical illnesses, volume overload is a complication of overzealous fluid therapy. Clinical signs of fluid overload include tachycardia, hypertension, breathlessness, dependent edema, and jugular venous distention. The end result of fluid overload is pulmonary edema. When symptoms of fluid overload are mild, sodium and fluid restriction is usually adequate treatment; when symptoms are severe, a diuretic is indicated. If volume overload is associated with heart failure, digitalis or vasodilator therapy should be considered.

Potassium Deficits

Clinical signs of *hypokalemia* are muscle weakness, paralytic ileus, U-wave or other changes on the ECG, and ventricular irritability. Furthermore, hypokalemia can enhance the action of nondepolarizing muscle relaxants.

More common causes of potassium deficiency are prolonged parenteral fluid therapy with no added potassium, excessive gastrointestinal losses with inadequate replacement, and diuretic therapy. In the absence of acid-base disturbance, concentration of potassium in serum can be used as a guide to estimate potassium deficits. Normal serum potassium concentration is 3.5–5 mEq/L. With a serum potassium concentration of 3 mEq/L, total body deficit is approximately 100 mEq. Thereafter, another 200 mEq of potassium is lost from the body store for each 0.5-mEq/L drop in serum potassium concentration.

Treatment of hypokalemia should be directed toward elimination of the precipitating cause and replacement of known deficits. Normally the amount of potassium added to intravenous fluids should be limited to 40 mEq in each liter, and the rate of infusion should be limited to 20 mEq each hour. If a higher concentration or a faster rate of infusion is desirable, electrical activity of the heart should be monitored continuously by ECG during infusion.

Overzealous replacement therapy, renal failure, and increased tissue catabolism (e.g., due to burns or crush injuries) can cause *hyperkalemia*. Symptoms and signs of hyperkalemia are nausea and vomiting, abdominal colic, and diarrhea; ECG signs are peaking of T-wave, widening of QRS complex, S–T segment depression, and asystole. Several methods are available for the treatment of hyperkalemia. Administration of sodium bicarbonate will, by inducing metabolic alkalosis, redistribute potassium to intracellular sites. Insulin added to a glucose infusion will promote movement of potassium into cells. The cationic exchange resin sodium polystyrene sulfonate will remove potassium from the gastrointestinal tract when it is given orally or rectally. Furosemide, by promoting urinary excretion of potassium, also can return serum potassium concentration toward normal. If myocardial depression is a complication, calcium chloride can be used to antagonize the depressant effect of potassium on the heart. The recommended doses of these drugs are listed in Table 20–1. When renal failure is the cause of hyperkalemia, peritoneal dialysis or hemodialysis is indicated.

Acid-base Abnormalities

Abnormal fluid and electrolyte losses are almost always complicated by acid-base abnormalities. *Metabolic acidosis* may be due to excessive loss of alkali (e.g., diarrhea, ureterosigmoidostomy, and renal tubular acidosis), formation of lactic acid (e.g., severe dehydration and shock, hypoxemia), or presence of other organic acids (e.g., renal failure, diabetic ketosis, and methanol or salicylate intoxication). In metabolic acidosis due to excess loss of bicarbonate, the anion gap is normal; with other causes, anion gap exceeds 15 mEq/L. (Anion gap is obtained by subtracting the serum concentration of chloride and bicarbonate from that of sodium.) Treatment directed at correcting the precipitating cause is all that is required when metabolic acidosis is mild. Severe metabolic acidosis, however, should be corrected with intravenous sodium bicarbonate. Hypertonic sodium bicarbonate solution can

TABLE 20–1. DRUGS USEFUL IN THE TREATMENT OF HYPERKALEMIA

Drug	Dose and Route
Sodium bicarbonate	50–150 mEq IV
Insulin and glucose	10 U regular insulin in 500 ml of 10% dextrose IV over 1 h
Sodium polystyrene sulfonate	40–80 g/day orally or rectally
Furosemide	40–80 mg IV or orally
Calcium chloride	1 g IV over 10–15 min with electro-cardiographic monitoring

cause volume overload, and rapid correction of acidosis can lead to hypokalemia; therefore, it is usually not advisable to correct severe acidosis completely with a single dose. The following equation should be used to calculate the initial dose:

$$\frac{\text{Sodium bicarbonate}}{\text{required (mEq)}} = \text{Base deficit} \times \text{Body weight (kg)} \times 0.15$$

After this dose, the patient's condition should be reassessed and treatment revised accordingly.

Metabolic alkalosis may be due to excessive loss of acid (e.g., vomiting, continuous gastric suction, intestinal fistula) or ingestion of alkali (the milk-alkali syndrome). When circulating volume is contracted, renal conservation of sodium is accompanied by reabsorption of bicarbonate; when potassium depletion is severe, sodium is reabsorbed in exchange for hydrogen ions by the kidneys. Both are common causes of metabolic alkalosis in surgical patients. Treatment of metabolic alkalosis should include saline infusion to replace volume deficits and administration of potassium chloride.

Respiratory disturbance can also lead to acid-base abnormalities. Acute *respiratory acidosis* is always the consequence of hypoventilation (e.g., due to respiratory depression by anesthetic agents or to splinting of chest and abdomen). Treatment of acute respiratory acidosis should be directed at correcting the precipitating cause. If necessary tracheal intubation and controlled ventilation should be employed. Overzealous mechanical ventilation is the most common cause of acute *respiratory alkalosis*. Treatment should be aimed at reducing tidal volume and respiratory rate accordingly. Mechanical dead space can be used to reduce alveolar ventilation in cases in which a large tidal volume is desirable.

ONGOING LOSSES

Like pre-existing deficits, ongoing losses can be external and obvious or internal and occult. Ongoing external loss of fluid can be measured accurately by monitoring the patient's input and output. It is more difficult to estimate the volume of sequestered fluid or third-space loss. This volume is only a few hundred milliliters after minor operations (e.g., elective hernia repair or operations on head and neck), but it can be 3 liters or more after extensive dissections (e.g., pancreatectomy or repair of abdominal aortic aneurysm). Therefore it is important to monitor urine output and central venous or pulmonary capillary wedge pressure when third-space loss is anticipated to be great.

TABLE 20–2.   ELECTROLYTE CONTENTS OF ALIMENTARY FLUIDS*

ALIMENTARY FLUID	NA$^+$ (mEq/L)	K$^+$ (mEq/L)	CL$^-$ (mEq/L)	HCO$_3^-$ (mEq/L)
Gastric fluid	60 (10–115)	10 (0–30)	130 (10–155)	
Pancreatic secretion	140 (115–185)	5	75 (55–95)	115
Bile	145 (130–165)	5	100 (90–180)	35
Duodenal fluid	140	5	80	
Ileal fluid	140 (80–150)	5	105 (40–140)	30
Colonic fluid	60	30	40	

* These are average values; the normal range is shown in parentheses.

Solutions used to replace ongoing losses from the intestine should be chosen to reflect the composition of the lost fluids. The electrolyte contents of intestinal and other alimentary fluids are listed in Table 20–2. Sequestered fluids on the other hand have a composition similar to that of extracellular fluid. A balanced salt solution should be used to replace such losses.

GENERAL GUIDELINES FOR REPLACEMENT THERAPY

In order to maintain fluid and electrolyte balance, it is important to administer basal requirements, replace existing deficits, and

TABLE 20–3.   ELECTROLYTE CONTENTS OF PARENTERAL SOLUTIONS*

SOLUTION	NA$^+$ (mEq/L)	K$^+$ (mEq/L)	CA^{++} (mEq/L)	CL$^-$ (mEq/L)	LACTATE (mEq/L)
Lactated Ringer's	130	4	3	109	28
0.9% (normal) saline	154			154	
M/6 sodium lactate	167				167
0.45% saline	77			77	
0.3% saline	51			51	
0.2% saline	34			34	

* Hypotonic saline solutions usually come with 5% dextrose.

keep up with additional losses. Whether the patient is on the ward or in the operating room, it is only a matter of simple arithmetic to calculate the total amount of fluid and electrolytes required and to replace it with a combination of 5% dextrose and hypotonic or isotonic saline. The composition of some commonly used parenteral fluids is given in Table 20–3.

For the patient who is old and infirm or who has cardiac, renal, or hepatic disease, replacement of large pre-existing deficits should be more gradual. Only half the calculated deficit should be replaced initially. In order to prevent pulmonary congestion, it may be necessary to monitor central venous or pulmonary capillary wedge pressure while the deficit is being replaced. In these cases, the patient's clinical condition should be reassessed frequently and management should be revised accordingly.

Blood Transfusion in Surgical Patients

Transfusion (of lamb's blood into man) was pioneered by Richard Lower in 1667. Due to obvious dangers associated with heterologous transfusion it was abandoned as a means of treating hemorrhagic shock until the 19th century, when James Blundell reintroduced the concept of human blood transfusion (both homologous and autologous) as a method of replacing blood loss of postpartum hemorrhage. Nevertheless it took almost another 100 years for the technique to become safe, which it did after the discovery of ABO blood groups by Karl Landsteiner in 1900.

HOMOLOGOUS BLOOD TRANSFUSION

In a modern blood bank, whole blood is seldom available for transfusion; it is separated into its components to meet specific needs: to replace blood loss, to replenish plasma volume, and to correct coagulopathies.

Common Blood Products and Their Components

Whole Blood.   One unit of whole blood contains 450 ml of donor blood in 63 ml of citrate-phosphate-dextrose-adenine (CPDA-1) anticoagulant. It can be stored at 4° C for up to 35 days. Labile coagulation factors V and VIII are reduced.

Red Cell Concentrate.   Also known as packed cells, red cell concentrate is obtained from whole blood by removing 200 ml of plasma. One unit has a volume of 300 ml and a hematocrit of 75%. It can be stored at 4° C for up to 35 days.

Leukocyte-Poor Red Cells.   Leukocyte-poor red cells are also known as "buffy coat–poor packed cells." The white cell fraction of red cell concentrate is removed by centrifugation, sedimentation, washing, or filtering. One unit has a volume of 200 ml. It should be infused within 24 hours of preparation because of potential contamination during preparation.

Frozen Red Cells.   Prepared from units of whole blood, red cells may be stored in the frozen state for 10 years. After thawing and reconstitution in normal saline, 70% of the origin red cell mass remains.

Platelet Concentrate (from Random Donors).   One unit contains 60×10^9 platelets suspended in 50 ml of plasma. It may be stored at 22° C for up to 5 days. But individual units that are pooled before transfusion should be infused promptly.

Platelet Concentrate (Obtained by Apheresis).   Another type of platelet concentrate is obtained by apheresis with intermittent or continuous-flow centrifugation from a single donor. It contains $200–400 \times 10^9$ platelets suspended in 200–300 ml of plasma. It is stored at 22° C and has a shelf life of 5 days if prepared in a closed system, but only 1 day if prepared in an open system.

Stored Plasma.   Stored plasma is separated from whole blood within 72 hours of collection. One unit has a volume of 200 ml. It contains all coagulation factors except V and VIII and its shelf life is 35 days at 4° C.

Frozen Plasma.   One unit of frozen plasma has a volume of 200 ml and contains 50% of original factor VIII. Separated from whole blood and frozen within 24 hours of collection, its shelf life is 12 months at −30° C and 3 months at −20° C.

Fresh-Frozen Plasma.   When plasma is separated from whole blood and frozen within 12 hours of collection it is called "fresh-frozen plasma." One unit has a volume of 200 ml and contains all coagulation factors. Shelf life is 12 months at −30° C or 3 months at −20° C. It requires 20 minutes to thaw.

Cryoprecipitated Factor VIII.   Also known as "cryoprecipitated plasma protein fraction," cryoprecipitated factor VIII has approximately 100 units of factor VIII activity and 250 mg of fibrinogen in a volume of 5–10 ml per bag. Shelf life is 1 year at −30° C or 3 months at −20° C, and it requires 10 minutes to thaw.

Antihemophilic Factor.   Also known as coagulation factor VIII, antihemophilic factor is a lyophilized fractionated plasma product heat-treated to inactivate human immunodeficiency virus (HIV) and some hepatitis viruses. It must be reconstituted before being used.

Albumin.   Albumin is available as 50–100 ml of 25% solution and as 250–500 ml of 5% solution. HIV and hepatitis viruses are eliminated during pasteurization. Shelf life is 5 years at 4° C and 3 years at room temperature.

Therapeutic Uses of Homologous Blood Products

To Replace Blood Loss

Red cell concentrates have superseded whole blood as blood replacements. All healthy patients with a normal preoperative hemoglobin concentration can tolerate a 20% loss of blood volume, as long as circulatory volume is maintained normal with the infusion of a physiologic saline solution (e.g., lactated Ringer's solution, normal saline). If loss of blood volume exceeds 20%, the decision of whether to initiate transfusion or continue hemodilution depends on the clinical condition of the patient. Packed cells are used to replace red cell loss. Since plasma is also lost, red cell concentrates should be reconstituted with normal saline, 5% albumin, or plasma (discussed in the next two sections). Reconstitution also reduces the viscosity and improves the flow characteristics of these red cell preparations.

Like red cell concentrates, leukocyte-poor red cells are also available for blood replacement. They should be used only for patients with a known transfusion reaction to white cells, for organ transplantation candidates, and for patients who require repeated transfusions. Frozen red cells, on the other hand, are costly to process. They are reserved for autologous transfusion only in persons with rare blood types or multiple red cell antibodies and in those for whom homologous transfusion is contraindicated (e.g., bone marrow transplant patients).

To Replenish Plasma Volume

As was pointed out in the previous section, infusion of a crystalloid solution may be used to sustain normal blood volume during the initial phase of hemorrhage. Since some of the infused saline solution will leave the intravascular space, it is generally recommended that 3 volumes of crystalloid be used for each volume of whole blood lost. When blood loss exceeds 20% of blood volume, replacement of subsequent plasma loss with a colloid solution is required to maintain oncotic pressure. Both 5% albumin and stored plasma are appropriate, unless replenishment of clotting factors is necessary. These products are also used to replace protein and fluid loss in victims of extensive burns. Five-percent albumin has many advantages over stored plasma; it is free of potential contamination by HIV and hepatitis viruses, is compatible with all blood groups, and has a long shelf life at room temperature.

To Correct Coagulopathies

Different blood products are used to correct specific coagulation defects. Stored plasma has all the plasma proteins except labile clotting factors V and VIII. It is indicated for replacing stable clotting factors and for rapid reversal of the anticoagulant effects of coumadin-like drugs. Fresh frozen plasma, on the other hand, has all the clotting factors intact. During massive transfusion, when a volume equal to or greater than the patient's blood volume must be replaced in less than 24 hours, red cells should be reconstituted with fresh-frozen plasma and stored plasma alternately, to avoid dilutional coagulopathy.

Platelet concentrates are used to treat thrombocytopenia due either to intrinsic illness (e.g., idiopathic thrombocytopenic purpura) or to dilutional coagulopathy during massive transfusion. In general 6 random donor units are given at a time to adult patients to raise the platelet count above the hemostatic level of 50,000/mm³. Ideally only platelet concentrates from donors with the ABO blood group identical to that of the recipient should be used, but this is not absolutely necessary. In some patients, HLA compatibility is an important consideration (e.g., in patients who had repeated transfusions and in bone marrow transplant recipients). In these instances platelet concentrates prepared by apheresis from HLA-matched donors can be used.

Cryoprecipitated factor VIII is used to treat bleeding diathesis in hemophilia A (classic hemophilia) and von Willebrand's disease. The factor VIII activity of an adult patient is increased by approximately 2% for each bag of cryoprecipitated factor VIII administered. Enough should be given to raise the activity level to 30% of normal in order to treat or prevent minor hemorrhage, to 50% to prevent hemorrhage following minor operations, and to 75% to prevent hemorrhage following major procedures. Ideally units from donors with the identical ABO blood group to that of the recipient should be used, but this is not absolutely necessary. Owing to its high fibrinogen content, this preparation can also be use for fibrinogen replacement. Unlike cryoprecipitated factor VIII, the antihemophilic factor preparation does not have the von Willebrand's factor and is suitable for treating only hemophilia A. It is heat-treated to inactivate all the HIV and some of the hepatitis viruses. It is the preferred product for repeated transfusion in hemophiliacs.

Homologous Blood Transfusion Reactions

Despite advances in testing of blood groups and subtypes and in fractionation and storage of blood components, transfusion reactions still occur in approximately 3% of the units of blood transfused. The recipient can react to both the formed elements and the soluble proteins of the donor's blood. Although ABO-incompatible or RH-incompatible transfusion reactions are potentially fatal, reactions to other blood or plasma proteins are less serious.

Febrile Reactions

Febrile reactions occur in 1–2% of all transfusions. A transfusion-related fever may be due to lysis of incompatible red cells or to reaction to white cells and other proteins. The latter is more common and can be prevented by the use of leukocyte-poor red cells or washed red cells.

Allergic Reactions

Development of mild urticaria during transfusion is as common as febrile reactions. This can be treated or prevented with administration of an antihistamine (chlorpheniramine, 10 mg given intravenously with each unit of blood but not exceeding 40 mg in 24 hours). On rare occasions bronchospasm, angioneurotic edema, and frank anaphylaxis are seen, particularly in recipients with strong anti-IgA antibodies. If the reaction is severe, the transfusion should be stopped and complications should be treated with epinephrine, bronchodilators, antihistamines, steroids, and other supportive measures. IgA-free blood should be requested for these persons in future transfusions.

Acute Hemolytic Transfusion Reactions

Acute hemolytic transfusion reactions are the consequence of lysis of the donor's red cells by the recipient's serum due to ABO or Rh incompatibility. Renal failure and disseminated intravascular coagulation are the most serious complications of incompatible blood transfusion. The immediate clinical signs of a reaction are chills, pyrexia, headaches, paresthesia, restlessness, nausea and vomiting, chest pain, shortness of breath, tachycardia, and hypotension. Most of these signs are masked in the anesthetized surgical patient, except cyanosis, hypotension, and general oozing at the surgical site. Treatment should include the following measures:

1. Stop infusing the incompatible blood immediately and send the unused fraction back to the blood bank for examination. (If the patient still requires blood, use compatible blood when it becomes available.)
2. Increase the inspired oxygen fraction.
3. Treat bronchospasm.
4. Support the circulation.
5. Monitor urine output and induce diuresis.
6. Monitor coagulation function and treat disseminated intravascular coagulation.

Delayed Hemolytic Transfusion Reactions

In patients who were exposed and sensitized to red cell antigens of minor subgroups in previous transfusion, the serum may be found to be compatible with red cells having these same antigens in a subsequent crossmatch. But following transfusion, a rapid rise in antibody titer can develop in the next few days, leading to lysis of transfused red cells. This delayed reaction is usually mild. Some reactions cause few symptoms; others can present as fever or prehepatic jaundice.

Other Complications of Homologous Blood Transfusion

Dilutional Coagulopathy

Stored blood is low in platelets and factors V and VIII. In massive transfusion, depletion of these factors can cause a significant bleeding diathesis. It can usually be prevented by transfusing 2 units of fresh-frozen plasma and 6 random donor units of platelet concentrates for every 10 units of blood given.

Hepatitis

The incidence of viral hepatitis in recipients following massive transfusion of stored blood was as high as 32% until the practice of testing all blood donors for hepatitis B surface antigen was introduced. The incidence of this complication has fallen dramatically; however transmission from carriers of non-A and non-B viral hepatitis remains a significant risk.

Acquired Immunodeficiency Syndrome

Please refer to "Blood Transfusion and AIDS" in Chapter 25.

Other Infectious Diseases

In addition to hepatitis B surface antigen and HIV antibodies, all donated blood is screened for syphilis infection. Nevertheless banked blood is a potential medium for transmission of infectious diseases, including cytomegalic and Epstein-Barr virus infection and malaria. But these incidents are relatively uncommon if donors are carefully selected.

Potassium Intoxication

Potassium diffuses out of red cells as stored blood ages. The potassium concentration of 35-day-old stored blood may be as high as 25 mEq/L. These potassium ions are recaptured by the red cells when they have regained their metabolic function. Therefore hyperkalemia is not seen in the recipient even after transfusion of a large volume of stored blood. During rapid transfusion this high potassium concentration of stored blood can cause myocardial depression and cardiac standstill during its first pass through the coronary circulation. Furthermore, stored blood is low in calcium ion concentration and is cold; these characteristics can aggravate the myocardial depressant effect of a high potassium concentration.

CITRATE INTOXICATION

Stored blood is prevented from coagulating by adding a CPDA-1 solution to remove calcium ions. Owing to an excess of citrate, hypocalcemia is a potential complication following massive transfusion of whole blood or stored and frozen plasma. Fortunately citrate is metabolized rapidly by the liver. A large drop in serum calcium ion concentration is unlikely, unless whole blood or plasma is administered at a rapid rate or the recipient is hypothermic. It is recommended that 500 mg of calcium gluconate or chloride should be given for every 2 units of whole blood or plasma transfused if it is given at a rate of 1 unit every 5 minutes or faster.

HYPOTHERMIA

Rapid transfusion of a large volume of cold stored blood can cause a large drop in body temperature, particularly in the anesthetized patient. Hypothermia involving the body core or the myocardium locally is a contributing factor in many reported cases of cardiac arrest associated with massive transfusion. Hypothermia can be alleviated by warming stored blood as it is being infused.

A PRACTICAL GUIDE TO CLINICAL TRANSFUSION

Before giving blood products to a patient, certain procedures should be strictly followed, so that an incompatible transfusion can be avoided. These procedures include determining the recipient's blood group, selecting donor blood that is compatible, testing for compatibility between the donor's red cells and recipient's serum, and verifying the identity of the recipient before transfusion. Since blood and plasma products (except platelet concentrates) deteriorate rapidly at room temperature, they should be stored properly before use.

Blood Group Testing and the Crossmatch

Determination of blood group involves testing the recipient's red cells for A, B and Rh antigens and screening the serum for most, but not all, of the irregular blood group antibodies. Crossmatch implies checking compatibility of the donor's red cells against the recipient's serum. A full crossmatch requires 1–1½ hours. A short crossmatch requires only 15–30 minutes, but the test is less sensitive. In most situations a full crossmatch should be routine, but an abbreviated crossmatch can be requested if blood is required urgently. In some life-threatening situations, blood transfusion may be necessary without a crossmatch. In the face of such a grave emergency, the patient's blood group and type should be determined, and group-specific blood (i.e., group- and type-identical blood) can be used for immediate transfusion. The routine use of O negative blood (blood from so-called universal donors) should be discouraged because some group O blood contains potent anti-A and anti-B antibodies that can destroy the red cells of recipients whose blood group is A, B, or AB.

Identifying the Recipient

Incompatible transfusions are usually the result of clerical rather than technical error. Properly identifying both blood products to be used and the recipient is the only way to avoid a mistake. The patient's name and hospital number on the label of the blood or plasma pack should match those on the patient's chart and identification bracelet; group and type of the donor's blood should match the recipient's. This checking procedure should be witnessed by one other responsible hospital staff member. Only properly labeled blood or plasma products should be accepted.

Storage of Blood Products

Blood products are expensive, even with a voluntary donor service. In order to avoid deterioration, whole blood, red cell concentrates, and plasma should be stored at 4° C in a nearby thermostatically regulated refrigerator until used. If the container bag of the product has been entered during preparation, it is potentially contaminated and should be infused when processed. Activity of labile clotting factors in thawed fresh-frozen plasma as well as that of cryoprecipitated factor VIII preparations and function of platelets in pooled concentrates deteriorate rapidly. These products should be infused as soon as they are prepared.

Infusion Sets and Filters

A disposable infusion set with an in-line filter should be standard equipment for infusing blood or plasma products. When whole blood or red cell preparations are infused, use of an 18-gauge or larger intravenous cannula is recommended so that an acceptable infusion rate can be achieved. Before and after the infusion of blood, the infusion set should be flushed with normal saline. Not all intravenous solutions are compatible with stored blood. The calcium in lactated Ringer's solution can promote clotting, and solutions containing glucose or dextran can cause rouleau formation.

In-line filter has a pore size of 80–175 μm. It removes larger cellular debris and clots and should be used for infusion of all blood and plasma products, including platelet concentrates. Since fibrinous clots trapped by the filter provide a good culture medium for bacteria, the infusion set and its filter should be discarded after transfusion is complete.

Several disposable microfilters with pore size of 10–40 μm are available, which remove microscopic cellular aggregates believed to be the cause of post-transfusion respiratory insufficiency. Because these filters trap a significant amount of platelets they should not be used during platelet transfusion. Furthermore, the ability of these filters to reduce the incidence of post-transfusion respiratory insufficiency is largely unproved. These filters are indicated only for high-volume transfusions or for patients with pre-existing pulmonary disease.

Blood Warmers

Incorporation of a blood-warming device in the infusion line eliminates complications associated with the use of cold stored blood during massive and rapid transfusion. Warming of blood can be achieved with a thermostatically controlled water bath or dry bath. In order to avoid damage to red cells and plasma proteins, the temperature of the bath should be kept at 37° C. The practice of prewarming blood in an oven is not recommended.

Infusion Rate

Infusion rate is largely determined by the nature of the problem that necessitates the transfusion. In most cases, transfusion of a unit of blood should be completed within 4 hours, but patients with cardiac disease may not tolerate transfusion of blood even at this slow rate. In order to avoid fluid overload in these patients, pretreatment with a diuretic should be considered.

Transfusion under pressure to increase the infusion rate is necessary for patients who are bleeding actively. This can be achieved by applying pressure to the plastic bag with an inflatable compressor or by using a hand pump in the infusion set. Injection of air into the container to achieve pressurization is absolutely contraindicated. It should be remembered that a large-bore intravenous cannula will do more to improve infusion rate than high pressure.

AUTOLOGOUS BLOOD TRANSFUSION

Autologous blood transfusion involves collecting the patient's blood and reinfusing it when required. Three methods, practiced independently or in combination with one another, are available to surgical patients: predeposition of blood before elective surgery, preoperative phlebotomy and hemodilution, and intraoperative blood salvage. Autologous transfusion is complementary to but does not supplant the use of homologous blood products.

Predeposition of Blood

Most blood bank facilities will accept predeposition of autologous blood for use in elective surgical procedures provided that significant blood loss is anticipated and that the patient-donor meets the following criteria:

1. Has a hemoglobin concentration of at least 11 g/dl and a hematocrit of 34% before each phlebotomy.

2. Is free of cardiorespiratory or other systemic disease that makes blood donation unsafe.

3. Tests negative for hepatitis B surface antigen, HIV antibodies, and syphilis. (To accept seropositive blood would expose blood bank personnel and hospital staff to the risk of infection and the possibility of contaminating homologous products inadvertently.)

Arrangements can also be made for designated donors to deposit homologous blood based on the same criteria. No age criterion is set for predeposition of blood. Obviously the volume collected should be proportional to the size of the child.

Since blood anticoagulated with CPDA-1 has a shelf life of 35 days at 4° C, weekly phlebotomy for 4 weeks up to 72 hours before the operation will make available 4 units of whole blood at the time of surgery. In the perioperative period, predeposited units are given as required in the order of collection, and unused units are redirected to join the homologous supply. All patient-donors in such a program are given oral iron supplements daily. That and the stimulus of repeated phlebotomy "prime" the bone marrow to produce red cells at an accelerated rate. This is an added advantage of blood predeposition before surgery.

Preoperative Phlebotomy and Hemodilution

In this technique phlebotomy is performed immediately before surgery but after induction of anesthesia. Up to 2 units of whole blood is collected from adults, and circulating volume is maintained normal by a continuous infusion of physiologic saline as blood is withdrawn. Like bank blood, the phlebotomized blood should be anticoagulated with CPDA-1 solution, not heparin. In the perioperative period, the collected blood is returned to the patient as required. The unit of diluted blood collected last is infused first. Unused units should not be redirected to the homologous supply.

Preoperative phlebotomy and hemodilution can be practiced on all healthy surgical patients with normal preoperative hemoglobin concentration and hematocrit if significant blood loss is anticipated during the procedure. This technique has several advantages:

1. Hemodilution decreases blood viscosity and improves microcirculation and tissue perfusion.

2. Loss of red cell mass is reduced during introperative bleeding.

3. Blood collected is fresh and all clotting factors are intact.

Intraoperative Blood Salvage

This technique involves collecting shed blood for reinfusion. The collected blood is simply filtered before retransfusion in the Bentley or Pleur-evac system; red cells are separated, washed, and resuspended in saline before reinfusion in the Cobe or Hemonetics system. The former is simple to operate but carries the risk of infusing cellular debris, platelet aggregates, activated coagulation factors, anticoagulants, free hemoglobin, and air into the patient with the salvaged blood. While the latter is free of the above complications, it requires expensive automated equipment and the attention of a full-time technician. The time required to process salvaged blood also means some delay in returning red cells to the patient. Neither method is suitable for salvage of blood in areas contaminated by sepsis or malignant cells.

Cardiopulmonary Resuscitation

The goal of cardiopulmonary resuscitation is to maintain ventilation, oxygenation, and circulation in basic life support and to improve ventilation and oxygenation and restore normal cardiac action and circulation in advanced life support. Standards in these techniques of life support were first published by the American Medical Association in 1974 and were updated in 1980, and again in 1986. They have also been adopted by national organizations in other countries. The recommendations are aimed at improving the efficiency of resuscitation and are not meant to restrain trained medical personnnel from acting in the best interests of the victim. These guidelines are summarized in the following sections.

BASIC LIFE SUPPORT

The state of consciousness of a victim who has collapsed suddenly should be determined immediately by the "shake and shout" maneuver. This consists of shaking the patient gently and calling out loudly to him. Once unresponsiveness has been established, the patient should be placed in the supine position and the ABCs of life support—airway, breathing, and circulation—should be instituted.

Airway

Obstruction of the upper airway by the tongue lying against the posterior pharyngeal wall is a common problem in supine, unconscious persons. Resuscitation will fail unless the obstruction is relieved. Two methods are now recommended to keep the airway open. In the *head tilt-chin lift* method, the rescuer extends the victim's head with one hand while supporting the chin and lifting it forward with the other (Fig. 22–1A). In the *jaw thrust* method,

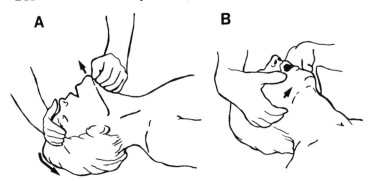

FIGURE 22–1. Methods of keeping the airway open: *A*, the head tilt-chin lift method, *B*, the jaw thrust method.

the jaw is thrust forward by simply grasping the angle of the victim's mandible on either side and displacing it anteriorly (Fig. 22–1*B*). Without head tilt, jaw thrust alone is the safer method of maintaining a patent upper airway in patients with suspected fracture of the cervical spine. Both methods require the rescuer to retract the victim's lower lip with the thumb.

Breathing

To date, no hepatitis B or HIV infection contracted through mouth-to-mouth resuscitation has been documented, but exposure to these infectious diseases is a potential risk to all health care personnel. In health care institutions, availability of masks and artificial airways equipped with one-way valves and disposable bag-and-mask units can minimize such exposure.

Once a patent airway is established, the rescuer should assess quickly whether the patient is breathing spontaneously by listening for breath sounds, feeling for the flow of air near the victim's nose and mouth, and observing the chest for respiratory movements. If spontaneous respiration is absent, artificial ventilation is indicated.

To perform *mouth-to-mouth ventilation* the rescuer should hold the victim's head and neck in one of the postures described above and pinch the victim's nose with one hand. Next, two large breaths should be delivered, to be followed by one full breath every 5 seconds if the victim is apneic but has a pulse. If the victim is also pulseless, two full breaths should be delivered for every 15 chest compressions in a single-rescuer resuscitation and one full breath for every five chest compressions in a two-rescuer operation (see below). Signs of adequate artificial ventilation are rise and fall of the victim's chest and escape of gas through the victim's mouth and nose during expiration. In addition, the rescuer should feel the resistance and compliance of the victim's lungs as they fill during the applied breaths.

Mouth-to-nose ventilation may be more effective than mouth-to-mouth ventilation in some patients, and *mouth-to-stoma ventilation* should be performed in patients who have a permanent tracheostomy. When the tracheostomy is only temporary, obstruction of the victim's mouth and nose is necessary if the tracheostomy tube does not have an inflatable cuff.

Improper head tilt-chin lift or jaw thrust is the most common cause of difficulties with ventilation. If mouth-to-mouth or mouth-to-nose ventilation is unsuccessful despite a properly opened airway, the victim's pharynx should be explored for secretions or foreign bodies. In the *finger sweep maneuver*, the victim remains supine. Forcing the victim's mouth open and grasping and lifting his tongue and jaw with one hand, the rescuer should run the index finger of the other hand down one side of the victim's mouth, across the back of the victim's throat, and up the other side of the victim's mouth in one sweeping motion. If this maneuver fails to extract the foreign body, subdiaphragmatic abdominal or chest thrusts should be applied. Both are designed to dislodge impacted foreign bodies.

In performing the *subdiaphragmatic abdominal thrust (Heimlich maneuver)* for unconscious victims, the rescuer kneels astride and faces the supine victim. With the heel of one hand placed against the victim's epigastrium at a site well below the rib cage and the other hand directly on top of the first, he or she presses into the victim's abdomen with an upward thrust using the entire body weight. The technique of *chest thrust* is similar to that of external chest compression (see "Circulation" below). This maneuver is reserved for morbidly obese patients and women in late stages of pregnancy. The sequence of thrust-finger sweep-ventilation described above should be repeated until the foreign body is removed and artificial ventilation can be carried out successfully.

Circulation

The third component of basic life support is assessment and support of the circulation. Absence of a palpable pulse in a major artery (carotid or femoral artery) is the cardinal sign of cardiac arrest. Both artificial ventilation and *external chest compression* are necessary in this emergency.

The victim should lie supine on a firm surface when external chest compression is performed. The rescuer should kneel at the victim's side and should place the heel of one hand over the lower half of the victim's sternum along its long axis and one finger-breadth cephalad to the xiphisternal junction. The other hand is placed on top of the first. With fingers interlocked, arms straight, and shoulders directly over the victim's sternum, the rescuer should apply sufficient pressure vertically downward to depress the sternum 4–5 cm (1½–2 in). Relaxation should follow compression, but the hands should not be removed from the victim's chest. It is recommended that the duration of compression should equal that of relaxation. In a one-rescuer operation, 15 external chest compressions should be delivered for every two full breaths; and in a two-rescuer operation, five chest compressions for every full breath. Contrary to previous recommendations, chest compressions should be performed at a rate of 80–100 times per minute.

Chest compression should be done smoothly and rhythmically. When properly done, external chest compression can generate systolic pressure of more than 100 mm Hg and mean pressure of 40 mm Hg in the carotid arteries.

Techniques in Infants and Children

The principles of basic life support in infants and children are similar to those recommended for adults. Owing to the discrepancy in size, however, modifications of the techniques described above are necessary:

1. An exaggerated head tilt is not necessary in infants and small children. The head should be held in a neutral position when opening of the airway is attempted in this group of patients.

2. In infants and small children, *mouth-to-mouth and nose ventilation* may be more appropriate than mouth-to-mouth or mouth-to-nose technique. Children need a smaller tidal breath than adults and volume should be guided by movement of the chest wall. Delivery of excessively large tidal volumes can lead to insufflation of air into the stomach and gastric distention.

3. Methods for removing foreign bodies from the airway of children are different from those recommended for adults. An object should be retrieved under direct vision and not by blind finger sweep, because the latter can force the foreign body deeper into the airway. Back blows together with chest thrusts is the method of choice to dislodge an impacted foreign body in infants under 1 year of age. *Back blows* are delivered with the heel of the hand aimed at the interscapular area while the victim straddles the rescuer's arm (Fig. 22–2A), and chest thrusts are applied with the infant lying head down across the rescuer's thigh. The sequence involves four back blows and four chest thrusts, to be followed by inspection of the mouth for foreign body and renewed attempts to ventilate the lungs. This sequence of blows, thrusts, ventilation should be repeated until the foreign body is removed and artificial ventilation is successful. In older children, subdiaphragmatic abdominal thrusts described for adults replace back

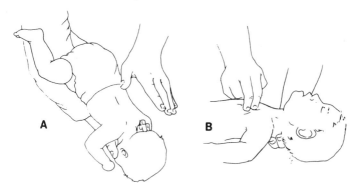

FIGURE 22–2. Basic life support in infants and children. *A*, Applying back blows to the infant. *B*, Applying chest compression to the infant. (From: Basic life support in infants and children. JAMA 244: 472, 1980.)

blows and chest thrusts as the method to dislodge impacted foreign bodies.

4. The brachial and femoral arteries are more accessible to palpation than the carotid arteries in young children.

5. Since the heart is higher in the rib cage in young patients, external chest compression should be applied with two or three fingers at a site one fingerbreadth below an imaginary line joining the nipples of infants (Fig. 22–2*B*) and at the lower half of the sternum in children. Depressing the sternum for 1.5–2.5 cm ($\frac{1}{2}$–1 in) is effective in infants, but a depression of 2.5–4 cm (1–1$\frac{1}{2}$ in) is required in children. In older children, the heel of the hand instead of the fingers should be used for external chest compression.

6. During cardiac arrest, external chest compression should be applied at a rate of 100/min in infants and 80–100/min in children. The ratio of compression to ventilation is always 5:1.

ADVANCED LIFE SUPPORT

"Advanced life support" refers to techniques aimed at improving ventilation and oxygenation of the victim and at diagnosing and treating the underlying rhythm disturbance during cardiac arrest. Advanced life support requires special equipment and drugs. It must be emphasized that basic life support should begin immediately when the diagnosis of respiratory or cardiac arrest is made and should be continued until the means of advanced life support become available.

Equipment

Within the hospital, equipment and drugs for advanced life support are usually stored on mobile carts stationed in strategic areas, including the operation suite and the recovery room. Equipment on these carts should include oxygen cylinders, pharyngeal airways, masks, a bag and valve assembly for ventilation of the lungs, endotracheal equipment, pharyngeal suction equipment, intravenous equipment, ECG monitor, and a direct current defibrillator. As soon as the cart arrives, the victim's oropharynx is cleared of secretions by suction, a pharyngeal airway is inserted, and ventilation with pure oxygen using a bag-valve-mask assembly is instituted. In addition, a bedboard should be placed under the victim. Except for momentary interruptions during defibrillation or other essential procedures, ventilation and chest compression should continue at the rates described for basic life support. At the first convenient moment, the victim's trachea should be intubated with a cuffed endotracheal tube, which protects the airway from contamination by stomach contents and eliminates the risk of inflating the stomach. The patient should be attached to the ECG monitor as soon as possible, and an intravenous infusion should be set up for drug administration. Cannulation of the internal jugular or subclavian vein is the method of choice unless it is contraindicated. If venous access is not immediately available, the following drugs can be given through the endotracheal tube if necessary: lidocaine, epinephrine, and atropine.

All the accessories for advanced life support are either immediately available or already attached to the patient in the operating room. Therefore resuscitation in this setting can begin as advanced life support. Administration of all anesthetic drugs should be discontinued; 100% oxygen should be delivered to the anesthetic circuit; the patient's ventilation should be controlled manually and not mechanically, so that it can be coordinated with chest compression. Malfunction of anesthesia equipment is always a potential cause of cardiac arrest in the operating room and must be ruled out as soon as possible.

Drugs

Atropine.   Atropine is a vagolytic agent capable of increasing the rate of discharge of the sinus node and of enhancing atrioventricular conduction. It is useful for treating sinus bradycardia, asystole, or atrioventricular block at the nodal level. The dose for bradycardia is 0.5 mg intravenously, and the dose for asystole is 1 mg intravenously. These doses may be repeated every 5 minutes, but the total dose should not exceed 2 mg in adults. (The vagolytic dose of atropine can be calculated in children according to body weight [0.02 mg/kg], but the single-bolus dose should not be less than 0.1 mg for young infants and not more than 1 mg for older children. This dose may be repeated in 5 minutes, but the total dose should not exceed 1 mg for children or 2 mg for adolescents.)

Bretylium.   Bretylium tosylate has a biphasic action on peripheral sympathetic function: an initial release of catecholamine is followed by postganglionic adrenergic blockade. It is used as an adjunct to treating ventricular fibrillation when lidocaine and defibrillation have failed. The initial dose is 5 mg/kg, to be followed by defibrillation. If fibrillation persists or recurs, 10 mg/kg followed by defibrillation may be repeated at 15–30 minute intervals. The total dose of bretylium tosylate should be limited to 30 mg/kg. (Dosage of bretylium tosylate in children is similar to that in adults.)

Calcium.   Calcium has only a limited role in cardiopulmonary resuscitation: to treat hypocalcemia and to counteract the effects of hyperkalemia and calcium channel blocker toxicity. Calcium chloride, 2–4 mg/kg, is the preferred preparation. Equivalent doses of calcium glucceptate or gluconate can also be given.

Epinephrine.   Epinephrine is a naturally occurring catecholamine with both alpha- and beta-agonist activities. It can convert ventricular asystole to ventricular fibrillation, increase the intensity of ventricular fibrillation, and lower the threshold of defibrillation. The recommended dose is 0.5–1 mg intravenously in adults, which is repeated every 5 minutes when necessary. In the absence of an intravenous infusion, epinephrine may be instilled into the tracheobronchial tree via an endotracheal tube or injected directly into the cardiac chamber; however, use of the intracardiac route should be reserved for dire emergencies, and only trained personnel should attempt this technique. (The dose of epinephrine in children is 0.01 mg/kg. It should be repeated every 5 minutes when required.)

Isoproterenol.   Isoproterenol is a synthetic, beta-adrenergic agonist with both chronotropic and inotropic properties. Given normally as an intravenous infusion, it is indicated for the treatment of atropine-resistant bradycardia. The dose is 2–10 μg/min in adults and should be adjusted according to its effect. (The dose is 0.1–1 μg/kg/min in children.)

Lidocaine.   In therapeutic concentrations, lidocaine reduces ventricular irritability and raises the fibrillation threshold without affecting myocardial contractility and atrioventricular conduction. It is particularly effective in treating ventricular arrhythmias following defibrillation or in suppressing ventricular irritability that ends in fibrillation after a successful defibrillation. The dose is 1 mg/kg given as a bolus intravenously. Additional boluses of 0.5 mg/kg may be given every 8–10 minutes to a total dose of 3 mg/kg. After successful defibrillation, a maintenance infusion of 20–50 μg/kg/min is recommended. In order to avoid systemic toxicity, blood level should be monitored and the dose adjusted after 24 hours. (The initial dose of lidocaine in children is also 1 mg/kg. If ventricular irritability continues to be a problem, this dose may be repeated to be followed by an infusion of 20–50 μg/kg/min.)

Sodium Bicarbonate. The role of sodium bicarbonate, a buffer base, in cardiopulmonary resuscitation is being challenged. Respiratory acidosis can be controlled by adequate alveolar ventilation, and metabolic acidosis by effective circulation through chest compressions. There are no convincing data to show that sodium bicarbonate is necessary if the ABCs of life support are carried out properly. Furthermore doses recommended in previous guidelines deliver a significant osmotic and sodium load to the patient's circulation. It is indicated only if a large base deficit is demonstrated by arterial blood gas analysis (see "Acid-Base Abnormalities" in Chap. 20); otherwise it should be given empirically only with discretion: not more than 1 mEq/kg initially and 0.5 mEq/kg for every 10 minutes of continued arrest thereafter. (In children the initial dose of sodium bicarbonate is 1 mEq/kg, but additional doses should be based on blood gas analysis.)

Other Drugs. In addition to the essential drugs mentioned above, many other cardiotropic and vasotonic agents are also useful during cardiopulmonary resuscitation: *procainamide, propranolol*, and *verapamil* for cardiac arrhythmias; *digoxin* for atrial flutter or fibrillation; *norepinephrine* and *metaraminol* for their pressor effects; *dopamine, dobutamine*, and *amrinone* for their inotropic action; *sodium nitroprusside* and *nitroglycerin* for their vasodilator properties; and *furosemide* for its diuretic effect. The student is advised to review the use of these agents in a pharmacology textbook.

Specific Treatment of Cardiac Arrest

Ventricular fibrillation and *pulseless ventricular tachycardia* should receive the same treatment. When they are recognized on the ECG monitor, the rescuer should deliver a precordial thump, with the fleshy part of the fist aimed at the midportion of the victim's sternum if a defibrillator is not yet available (not indicated in children). This maneuver is often successful in restoring rhythmic cardiac activity. If it is not successful, artificial ventilation and chest compression are continued and electrical defibrillation is carried out with the arrival of the "arrest cart." The first attempt at defibrillation is made using 200 joules (2 joules/kg in children) with electrodes placed just to the right of the upper sternum and just below and to the left of the left nipple. A second attempt using 200–300 joules (4 joules/kg in children) should be made immediately if the first attempt fails. If this second attempt also fails, a third attempt using up to 360 joules should be made. Failure at this point requires administration of epinephrine, lidocaine, or bretylium before further attempts at defibrillation are made. (The dose of epinephrine is repeated every 5 minutes and each dose of lidocaine is followed by an attempt at defibrillation using up to 360 joules. If defibrillation is still unsuccessful after the maximum dose of lidociane has been given, bretylium tosylate is administered and each dose is followed by an attempt at defibrillation.) All the while, artificial ventilation and chest compression should not be interrupted except for brief moments during defibrillation. Adequate artificial ventilation and circulation will prevent the development of acidosis, but sodium bicarbonate may be considered after several failed attempts at defibrillation. (The initial energy level for defibrillation in children is 2 joules/kg. If this is unsuccessful, two subsequent attempts at 4 joules/kg should be made. If these are also unsuccessful epinephrine, lidocaine, or bretylium tosylate is given as indicated and attempts at defibrillation are repeated.)

Ventricular asystole (cardiac standstill) is a sign of prolonged myocardial hypoxemia, extensive ischemia, massive infarction, severe acidosis, or hyperkalemia. Occasionally a high vagal tone may be responsible for asystole. Confirmation of this lack of cardiac rhythm should be sought in two separate ECG leads. Resuscitation efforts include (1) effective ventilation and chest compression to reoxygenate the myocardium and to wash out toxic metabolites and (2) repeated doses of epinephrine and atropine as described. If asystole gives way to fibrillation, defibrillation is indicated. When these drugs are unsuccessful, sodium bicarbonate should be administered and transvenous or percutaneous pacing should be considered. Asystole due to a high vagal tone responds readily to atropine or other chronotropic agents, but cardiac standstill due to myocardial damage has a poor prognosis.

Besides ventricular fibrillation or asystole, arrhythmias that are causing circulatory failure should also be treated as cardiac arrest. The treatment of pulseless *ventricular tachycardia* has been described. Some patients with ventricular tachycardia have relatively normal blood pressure and few symptoms. If cardiac output is adequate, intravenous lidocaine should be given. Procainamide is a second-line drug that may be employed. When ventricular tachycardia is resistant to antiarrhythmic therapy or when the patient's blood pressure is labile, a direct current countershock timed to discharge approximately 20 msec after the intrinsic R-wave should be administered, starting with 50 joules and increasing the energy level to 100, 200, and up to 360 joules as required in adults. (For cardioversion in children use 0.2–1 joule/kg.) Torsade de pointes is a subtype of ventricular tachycardia, for which quinidine-like drugs are contraindicated and electrical pacing is the treatment of choice.

Paroxysmal supraventricular tachycardia that is not causing hemodynamic instability can be treated by invoking the vagal reflex (e.g., carotid sinus massage or Valsalva's maneuver) or with verapamil, digoxin, or beta-adrenergic antagonists. If it is unresponsive to these antiarrhythmic agents or if circulatory instability is present, synchronous cardioversion is indicated, starting with 75–100 joules and increasing the energy output to 200 and then 360 joules in subsequent attempts in adults. (In children use 0.2–1 joule/kg.) Overdrive pacing is an alternative to direct current cardioversion.

Bradycardia requires treatment only if there is hypotension or circulatory failure. *Sinus* or *junctional bradycardia* and *heart blocks* may respond to atropine or isoproterenol. Transvenous pacing is indicated if bradycardia persists or atrioventricular conduction is tenuous.

In *electromechanical dissociation* the heart has relatively normal electrical activity but no effective mechanical function. The underlying cause may be mechanical in origin (e.g., inadequate filling as in hypovolemia, outflow obstruction as in massive pulmonary embolus, and cardiac tamponade or cardiac rupture) or it may be myocardial ischemia or hypoxemia. Treatment should be directed at correcting the underlying cause. Electromechanical dissociation seen during cardiac arrest carries a grave prognosis. Effective ventilation and chest compression should be started without delay; epinephrine is indicated; and sodium bicarbonate may be considered.

Postresuscitation Care

The cause of cardiac or respiratory arrest should be sought and treated in all patients after resuscitation, but the type of general care that is required depends entirely on the outcome of resuscitation efforts. The patient who has no neurologic deficit and who is maintaining a normal blood pressure without arrhythmias needs only intensive monitoring and continuing observation of circulatory, respiratory, cerebral, renal, and hepatic function. The patient who has single- or multiple-system failure requires ventilatory or circulatory support, antiarrhythmic therapy, dialysis, or cerebral resuscitation.

The organ most susceptible to ischemic and hypoxemic injuries during cardiac arrest is the brain. One fifth of long-term survivors of cardiac arrest have neurologic deficits. If a patient remains unconscious, attempts should be made to preserve cerebral perfusion and oxygenation. These measures include the use of vasoactive agents to maintain normal systemic blood pressure, steroids to decrease cerebral edema, and diuretics to reduce intracranial pressure. Seizure activity should be controlled, supplemental oxygen should be given, and a moderate degree of hyperventilation is helpful ($PaCO_2$ of 25–35 mm Hg). Some authors also recommend barbiturate coma and moderate hypothermia, but the benefits of these treatment modalities are still controversial.

Decision to Terminate Resuscitative Efforts

All physicians are obliged to initiate cardiopulmonary resuscitation as soon as respiratory or cardiac arrest is diagnosed, but the victim's personal physician should be consulted before resuscitative efforts are discontinued. Unconsciousness, absence of spontaneous respiration and brainstem reflexes, and fixed dilated pupils lasting 15–30 minutes or longer indicate brain death unless the patient is hypothermic or is under the effects of barbiturates or under general anesthesia. However, unresponsiveness of the heart to resuscitative measures, rather than clinical signs of brain death, is a better endpoint upon which to decide to terminate resuscitation. Absence of electrical activity of the heart (asystole) despite adequate resuscitative efforts usually means cardiac death.

Resuscitation of the Newborn

The neonate switches from placental to pulmonary respiration at birth. During this critical period many factors can cause hypoventilation, apnea, and circulatory insufficiency including the following:

1. Drugs administered to the mother (e.g., anesthetic agents, narcotic analgesics, sedatives, tranquilizers)
2. Neonatal asphyxia secondary to maternal hypotension or hypoxemia, placental insufficiency, compression of the umbilical cord, and difficult forceps delivery
3. Severe prematurity
4. Hypovolemia due to bleeding from the fetoplacental unit (e.g., placenta previa or abruptio placentae)
5. Birth injuries (e.g., pneumothorax, intracranial hemorrhage, fracture of the cervical spine)
6. Congenital abnormalities of the respiratory tract and the great vessels
7. Metabolic derangements (e.g., hypothermia, hypoglycemia).

TECHNIQUES OF CARDIOPULMONARY RESUSCITATION

Over 90% of all neonates make the transition to pulmonary respiration at birth without complications. However a significant number of the remainder need intensive resuscitation. Techniques for resuscitation are discussed in the next several sections, followed by a summary of assessment and management of newborns published by the American Medical Association in 1986.

Pulmonary Ventilation

Newborns who have depressed respiratory function and do not respond to tactile stimulation should receive positive-pressure ventilation via face mask. Fully extending the neck can cause airway obstruction in neonates, so the head should be kept in a neutral position when manual ventilation is attempted. An oropharyngeal airway is helpful in maintaining a patent airway, and an orogastric tube is advisable to decompress the stomach periodically.

Positive-pressure ventilation using bag and mask should be delivered to newborn infants at a rate of 40 breaths/min. A pressure of 30–40 cm of water may be required to initiate effective inflation of the lungs during the first few breaths. Thereafter peak airway pressure should be limited to 30 cm H_2O. Excessive airway pressure can cause pneumothorax or pulmonary gas leaks. Although the inspired atmosphere should be enriched with oxygen, pure oxygen is rarely required for prolonged periods. A PaO_2 of 150 mm Hg for 2 hours or more can cause retrolental fibroplasia, particularly in premature infants.

During ventilation of the lungs, chest expansion, breath sounds, heart rate, and color should be monitored. Most depressed neonates will respond to positive-pressure ventilation via a face mask. If improvement is not forthcoming, direct laryngoscopy and tracheal intubation are indicated.

The infant's larynx lies farther anterior and superior than the adult's. Direct laryngoscopy should be attempted with a straight blade (see "Techniques of Intubation" in Chap. 13). The endotracheal tube used should allow a small gas leak between it and the trachea when airway pressure reaches 10–15 cm H_2O. A 2.5-mm tube is recommended for infants who weigh less than 1 kg, a 3-mm tube for those weighing 1–2 kg, a 3.5-mm tube for those weighing 2–3 kg, and a 4-mm tube for those weighing over 3 kg. Positive-pressure ventilation via an endotracheal tube should be delivered at a rate of 40–60 breaths/min.

Under certain circumstances, the trachea of the newborn should be suctioned before the lungs are ventilated. These indications include frank vaginal bleeding during the second stage of labor and contamination of amniotic fluid by particulate meconium. (The presence of watery meconium alone does not require tracheal toilet.) Tracheal suctioning can be achieved by introducing an endotracheal tube for 1–2 cm below the vocal cords and then applying suction by mouth through a face mask as the endotracheal tube is withdrawn. After the blood clot or meconium is retrieved from the airway, the endotracheal tube should be left in place and the lungs should be ventilated as described.

Closed-Chest Compression

A heart rate consistently below 100/min in neonates is indicative of circulatory depression. The most common causes of circulatory failure are hypoxemia, hypercapnia, and metabolic acidosis. These asphyxiated infants will regain normal circulatory function when ventilation and oxygenation are restored. A heart rate below 60 beats/min is an indication for closed chest compression; so is a heart rate below 80 beats/min despite adequate ventilation. The two-handed chest-encircling method, in which the rescuer's hands encircle the chest of the infant with thumbs placed on the sternum at a point just below the level of the nipples, is the method of choice (Fig. 23–1). In premature infants the thumbs may have to be superimposed. In larger infants the two-finger technique described for pediatric patients may be indicated (see "Techniques in Infants and Children" in Chap. 22). The sternum should be depressed for 1.5–2 cm ($\frac{1}{2}$–$\frac{3}{4}$ in) at a rate of 120 times/min.

Correction of Hypovolemia

Hypovolemia should be suspected if the umbilical cord has been clamped early or if there is bleeding from the fetal-placental unit. It should be suspected also in the neonate who has been acidotic or who is not responding properly to resuscitation. The hypovolemic infant is pale and lethargic and has a prolonged capillary refill time, a thin thready brachial or femoral pulse, and low arterial and central venous pressure. It is difficult to measure arterial

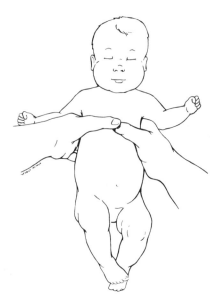

FIGURE 23–1. Chest compression in the neonate: the two-handed chest-encircling method.

pressure in neonates. Use of Doppler ultrasonography to measure systolic blood pressure (normally 50–70 mm Hg) is helpful. Cannulation of the umbilical artery allows direct pressure monitoring and sampling of blood for analysis of respiratory gases and pH determination. It is also a safe route of administration for fluid and drugs. Although the introduction of a catheter via the umbilical vein to measure central venous pressure (normally 4–12 cm water) is also helpful in an emergency, it is a potential source of infection and can cause portal vein thrombosis. The catheter should be removed at the end of resuscitation.

In the presence of hypovolemia, volume expansion can be achieved with 5% albumin, normal saline, or lactated Ringer's solution, or O negative blood with a low antibody titer cross-matched against maternal blood. Initially 10 ml/kg should be given, and it may be repeated when necessary.

Correction of Hypoglycemia

Hypoglycemia is a serious and not infrequent cause of neonatal depression. Premature infants and infants of diabetic mothers are especially at risk. This disorder should be corrected immediately by administering 2 mg/kg of 25% dextrose (mixed 50% dextrose with an equal volume of distilled water) to be followed by an infusion of 10% dextrose at a rate not exceeding 4 ml/kg/hr.

Drugs

Naloxone is a pure narcotic antagonist that has been found useful for reversing neonatal respiratory depression induced by narcotic analgesics given to the mother. The recommended dose, 10 μg/kg, can be given subcutaneously, intramuscularly, intravenously, or transtracheally and should be repeated when necessary. Since its duration of action is shorter than that of long-acting narcotic analgesics, continuing observation of the neonate is mandatory.

Epinephrine is indicated in cardiac standstill or when heart rate is below 80 beats/min despite adequate resuscitative measures. The recommended dose is 10–30 μg/kg, which can be given intravenously or transtracheally. This dose should be repeated every 5 minutes as necessary.

The usefulness of *atropine* and *calcium chloride* in neonatal resuscitation is being questioned. *Sodium bicarbonate*, on the other hand, is indicated only in the presence of severe metabolic acidosis despite adequate ventilation and chest compression (pH <7.00). Dose should be guided by the base deficit in arterial blood (see ''Acid-Base Abnormalities'' in Chap. 20). Both the 7.5% and 8.4% solutions are hypertonic and can cause rapid expansion of intravascular volume and intracranial hemorrhage in neonates.

They should be diluted with an equal volume of 5% dextrose or distilled water before they are given to neonates.

Vascular Access

An effective route for administration of drugs is important during resuscitation. Veins in the extremities are often accessible in neonates and should not be ruled out without careful inspection. Both naloxone and epinephrine are effective when given via the endotracheal tube; the calculated dose should be washed in with 1–2 ml of normal saline. Cannulation of the single thin-walled umbilical vein with a 3.5 or 5 F catheter is relatively easy. The tip of the catheter should be advanced to a point deep to the skin of the abdominal wall where free flow of blood is present. Cannulation of one of the two thick-walled umbilical arteries, on the other hand, is technically more difficult but is a safer route for administration of hypertonic solutions. (If an umbilical vein catheter is lodged inadvertently in the portal vein, infusion of hypertonic sodium bicarbonate may cause phlebitis and thrombosis of the portal circulation.) The arterial route also offers a conduit for pressure monitoring and sampling of blood for blood gas analysis.

A PRACTICAL GUIDE TO MANAGEMENT OF THE NEWBORN

During the second stage of labor, the mouth and nose of the neonate should be suctioned as soon as the head emerges. Successful passage of a suction catheter into the pharynx via the nose confirms the absence of choanal atresia. Immediately after birth, the cord should be clamped after it has stopped pulsating. Thereafter the infant should be placed naked with head down under a radiant heat lamp. He or she should be thoroughly dried with a towel to reduce heat loss through evaporation. The tactile stimulation of being dried will stimulate the baby to cry and initiate the first breath. Additional tactile stimulation — slapping the infant's sole or rubbing the back—may be necessary. Suction through the mouth and nose may be repeated at this stage. Since stimulation of the hypopharynx can cause reflex bradycardia, the heart rate should be monitored.

Assignment of Apgar scores at 1 minute and at 5 minutes after birth is the most widely accepted system of neonatal evaluation. In this system a score of 0, 1, or 2 is given to five objective signs: heart rate, respiration, muscle tone, reflex irritability, and color (Table 23–1). These scores should be documented regardless of resuscitative efforts. If the 5-minute score is below 7, assessment at 5-minute intervals should be continued until 20 minutes after birth.

TABLE 23–1.   THE APGAR SCORE

Signs	0	1	2
Heart rate	Absent	Below 100/min	Above 100/min
Respiration	Absent	Slow, irregular	Good, crying
Muscle tone	Limp	Some flexion of extremities	Active motion
Reflex irritability (to catheter in nares)	No response	Grimace	Cough, sneeze, cry
Color	Blue, pale	Pink body, blue extremities	Completely pink

Most babies will be crying and moving vigorously. They will look pink and have a heart rate well above 100 beats/min soon after birth (Apgar score of 8 or above). Such babies do not need resuscitation, but the stomach contents should be aspirated. A soft catheter attached to a syringe should be used. Successful introduction of the catheter into the stomach rules out esophageal atresia, and emptying of the stomach prevents regurgitation and aspiration. If more than 30 ml is aspirated, gastrointestinal obstruction should be suspected. Babies who remain stable at 5 minutes should be wrapped in a warm blanket and returned to the mother or placed in a bassinette.

If respiration is erratic or absent or if heart rate is less than 100 beats/min, resuscitative measures should be instituted as follows:

1. Clear the hypopharynx of secretions if necessary. (Suction should be effective but brief, so as not to interfere with ventilation.)

2. *If respiration is depressed but heart rate is 100 beats/min or above,* enrich the inspired atmosphere with 100% oxygen and continue to stimulate the baby gently. Give naloxone if narcotic analgesic given to the mother is the cause of hypoventilation. (Most such babies respond to these measures and have an Apgar score above 8 by 5 minutes.)

3. *If respiration is depressed and heart rate is between 60 and 100 beats/min* assist ventilation with bag and mask, using 100% oxygen. (Most such infants respond to ventilation and oxygenation by increasing heart rate to above 100/min, turning pink, and beginning to breathe normally.)

4. *If heart rate is below 60 beats/min OR if heart rate remains below 80 beats/min despite adequate ventilation* by face mask, intubate the trachea, assist ventilation, and initiate chest compression.

The most common cause of neonatal depression is asphyxia. Asphyxiated babies improve rapidly with adequate ventilation and oxygenation. If improvement does not follow institution of resuscitative measures, other casues of neonatal depression should be sought (e.g., hypovolemia, hypoglycemia, birth injury).

Anesthetic Mishaps, Quality Assurance, and Risk Management

The frequency of litigation associated with medical practice has increased sharply in recent years, both in North America and in Western Europe. The awards in many of the cases settled also have escalated dramatically, sometimes to amounts that were unthinkable just a few years ago. There are many reasons for these changes. Society today is better educated and has a greater abundance of material wealth than ever before. Not only is the general public increasingly aware of the progress in modern medicine, but many regard these advances as assurance of abundance in health. With rising expectations, demands for perfection in the results of care and treatment are only natural.

Administration of an anesthetic is a complex and demanding pursuit fraught with pitfalls and hazards. Anesthesia is a high-risk specialty, not least with regard to the potential for litigation. The anesthesiologist, being a member of the surgical team, may also be named in suits in which he or she has no direct responsibility. This chapter is not a dissertation on medical jurisprudence, but it focuses instead on safely conducted anesthesia, which reduces the opportunities for mishaps and thus the frequency of litigation.

Anesthetic Mishaps

It has been estimated that perioperative mortality attributable to anesthesia occurs at a rate of one per 10,000 anesthetics. However, there are no data on the prevalence of anesthetic accidents or the incidence of nonfatal anesthetic injuries. All anesthetic accidents have the potential to cause harm. Of all "critical incidents" 6.5% can be expected to be associated with unfavorable outcomes (death, cardiac arrest, cancelled procedure, and extra stay in recovery room, intensive care unit, or hospital).

When mishaps in the operating room are analyzed, certain recurring problems are identified:

1. Mistaken identity of the patient leading to incorrect operation or mismatched transfusion
2. Incorrect position of the patient on the operating table leading to nerve palsy or cardiovascular and respiratory embarrassment (see "Positioning the Patient on the Operating Table" in Chap. 15)
3. Misuse or malfunction of anesthetic equipment leading to asphyxia, barotrauma of the airway, and other injuries (Table 24–1)
4. Misuse or malfunction of electrical instruments leading to burns or electrocution
5. Complications associated with the use of intravenous equipment leading to misplaced catheters, embolization of catheter fragments, air embolism, and so forth

**TABLE 24–1.   MISHAPS ASSOCIATED WITH THE USE OF
ANESTHETIC EQUIPMENT**

Equipment	Possible Malfunction or Misuse
Anesthetic Machine	
Gas supply	Incorrect connection, leaks, empty cylinders, total disruption of pipeline supply
Flowmeters	Incorrect settings, leaks
Vaporizers	Wrong agent (a methoxyflurane vaporizer filled with halothane will deliver 10 times the concentration indicated on the dial), leaks, errors in calibration
Anesthetic Circuit	Disconnection, leaks, improper connection (especially with the circle system), improper setting of relief valve and safety pop-off valve leading to high airway pressure
Ventilator	Disconnection, leak, failure of changeover mechanism, loss of power
Ancillary Equipment	
Laryngoscope	Damage to teeth and lips, failure of light source (especially in an emergency such as rapid-sequence induction)
Endotracheal tube	Bronchial or esophageal intubation, leakage or rupture of cuff, disconnection, accidental extubation, obstruction (due to kinking, compression, herniated cuff)
Malleable stylet	Perforation of airway
Laryngeal spray	Systemic toxicity of local anesthetics
Suction apparatus	Failure (especially during an emergency)

6. Improper labeling of drugs, leading to administration of the wrong drug or gross overdose

7. Improper monitoring of the patient's condition and failure to recognize signs of impending danger.

It is rare that an isolated incident results in catastrophe. Although equipment malfunction appears to be involved in a large number of these accidents, there is almost always some degree of additional human error that compounds the problem. The human factor is commonly related to a lack of vigilance due to haste, fatigue, or distraction. Inexperience or inadequate knowledge about the equipment, technique, or procedure also has been found to contribute to disaster.

Prevention of Mishaps

It is agreed that many of the incidents described are avoidable. A concerted effort to reduce their occurrence requires that attention be focused on the patient, on the proper care and use of anesthetic and ancillary equipment, and on maintaining vigilance. The importance of properly identifying the patient and nature and site of the operation and of assessing the patient's medical condition has been discussed in previous chapters.

Proper Care and Use of Equipment. In a specialty such as anesthesiology where there is a broad interface between sophisticated technology and clinical methods, it is mandatory that the practitioner understand the principles and workings of the equipment he uses. Only equipment that meets current safety standards should be installed. When new standards are issued or old ones revised, the anesthesiologist has the responsibility of upgrading the equipment in his own institution. All incidents of malfunction or potential misuse should be reported immediately so that they can be acted upon and rectified without delay.

Although the function of all electrical instruments and anesthetic equipment is checked periodically by the technical staff of the hospital, it is the duty of the anesthesiologist to ensure that these devices are in satisfactory condition and functioning properly every time they are used. To do so the anesthesiologist should develop a checklist somewhat similar to those used by aircraft pilots for routine preflight equipment check. The checklist should be comprehensive enough for safe practice yet convenient enough for frequent use. The following suggested scheme can easily be incorporated into local routines. Items to be checked before each operation can be extended to include the patient and drugs.

PATIENT. Identity, nature and site of operation, consent, availability of blood, if applicable.

ANESTHETIC MACHINE. Gas supply (pipelines and cylinders), flowmeters, vaporizers, oxygen flush control, oxygen analyzer, alarm.

ANESTHETIC CIRCUIT.   Connection to machine, reservoir bag, relief (expiratory) valve, safety pop-off valve, leaks, specific components of individual circuits (e.g., soda-lime canister of the circle system, inner tubing of the Bain circuit).

VENTILATOR.   Inspiratory phase, changeover from inspiration to expiration, expiratory phase, changeover from expiration to inspiration.

ENDOTRACHEAL EQUIPMENT.   Laryngoscope (type and size of blade, light source); endotracheal tube (size, length, integrity of cuff); ancillary equipment (intubation forceps, malleable stylet, laryngeal spray, lubricant, cuff inflator).

SUCTION APPARATUS.   Source, tubing, and catheter.

INTRAVENOUS DRUGS.   Anesthetics, relaxants, narcotic analgesics, other drugs (e.g., vasopressors), correct labels.

In many ways the working environment of anesthesiologists is not conducive to safety. Unlike airplane pilots, they have yet to benefit from the consideration of ergonomic design in the operating room, but they can position themselves and their equipment to obtain a convenient view of the anesthetic machine, the monitors, and the patient and they should allow themselves sufficient space to operate efficiently. The work table and top of the anesthetic machine should be kept tidy. A neatly organized working environment minimizes distraction and decreases fatigue.

Vigilance and Diligence.   Vigilance is the key to successful monitoring. Although it is customary to record vital signs only every 5 minutes, it must be remembered that cerebral dysfunction and death can occur within 10 seconds and 4 minutes, respectively, after the onset of cerebral anoxia. Therefore some form of continuous monitoring of oxygenation (e.g., color of skin or shed blood, pulse oximetry) and cardiac output (e.g., heart sounds) is mandatory. (Pulse oximetry will do both and is the preferred method.)

Unfortunately eternal vigilance is not a human characteristic. It is often during the calm of the maintenance phase that distraction and fatigue become more evident and attention lapses. It is therefore not surprising that over half of reported mishaps occur during this period. In recognition of this problem, automated monitoring instruments with alarms have been introduced (see Chap. 14). Although these devices are undeniably useful, they are only aids, not substitutes for the discipline of vigilance. The diligence of the anesthesiologist is still required.

In the Event of Mishaps

The operating room environment is a critical area for mishaps. Most anesthesiologists will admit that they have experienced minor mishaps more than once in their career. How, then, should these mishaps be handled?

First and foremost, the situation should be corrected as rapidly and completely as possible and assistance should be summoned if the need arises. All that has taken place should then be documented very thoroughly at the earliest opportunity, though this may be difficult in the heat of the moment. A thorough documentation made at the time of the incident is of paramount importance if the anesthesiologist is unfortunate enough to be involved in litigation as a result of the misadventure. Memory for details is notoriously short.

At the postoperative visit, the anesthesiologist should explain to the patient, as fully as possible, the circumstances of the occurrence. This should be a complete and truthful explanation, with due respect and sympathy, so that the patient can understand exactly what has befallen him and yet have some insight into the anesthesiologist's difficulties. In most cases patients are not hostile and may even volunteer information concerning previously unrecognized predisposing factors that may absolve the anesthesiologist. The anesthesiologist can gain the respect of the patient by discussing the matter frankly.

If there is any possibility that legal action will follow, the anesthesiologist should contact his medical defense organization or insurance carrier as soon as possible. The serving of a writ and a statement of claim outlining the complaints of the injured party (the plaintiff) may be the first intimation that legal action is being taken. In this situation, it is imperative that the defense organization or insurance carrier be contacted immediately because the defendant's position may be jeopardized if this first action is not taken at the earliest opportunity.

The defense organization or insurance carrier will no doubt require complete details of the incident. The most important rule to follow in any episode is to be complete, in content and veracity, in the information that is given. It should be remembered that the legal process may move very slowly, so it may be years before a case comes before the courts. The parties concerned are rarely able to remember the details required of them if records are not available. If the details of a mode of treatment are not recorded, it may be assumed erroneously that the treatment was not given. Therefore impeccable record keeping can assist the defense considerably.

QUALITY ASSURANCE
AND RISK MANAGEMENT

It is obvious from previous sections that all health care institutions should set standards for anesthesia practice and direct efforts to prevent mishaps. The Joint Commission on Accreditation of Hospitals has ruled that all hospitals should establish quality assurance-risk management programs in clinical departments.

Quality assurance in the health care industry refers to a dynamic process by which standards of services in an institution are defined and achievement of these standards is assured by assessment of outcome. The goal of risk management is to prevent accidents and injuries and to cope with the consequences should they occur. These two processes are necessarily related: both involve detection, evaluation, and resolution of problems. While quality assurance defines the quality of care, risk management removes the potential to cause harm. Through prevention, risk management improves the quality of care.

To establish a quality assurance and risk management program, the department should establish policy and credential criteria for members of its staff, draw up procedural manuals and guidelines of safe practice, and set up audit and review committees. These committees should be concerned with issues in three areas: structure, process, and outcome. Structure refers to physical facilities and their utilization (e.g., availability of capnographs and pulse oximeters in the operating suite or duration of stay in the post-anesthesia care unit). Process is the way anesthesia is practiced by members of staff (e.g., completeness of record, compliance with monitoring guidelines). Outcome in anesthesia practice is measured by prevalence of critical incidents and anesthetic complications (e.g., accidental extubation, intraoperative hypotension and hypovolemia, perioperative deaths). When a problem is identified in any area, its implications are thoroughly assessed, corrective procedures are recommended and implemented, and progress is followed up and reevaluated at a later date.

A quality assurance and risk management program can be carried out successfully by a department only with the full cooperation of its staff. In order to encourage and foster honesty, the program must be nonthreatening to its participants. It should be made clear that documentations collected for the purpose of quality assurance cannot be used as evidence in a lawsuit. (In the United States such data are protected by peer review legislation.) Quality assurance activities should not be used as a yardstick for career advancement, nor should disciplinary actions result directly from them.

AIDS and the Anesthesiologist

Acquired immunodeficiency syndrome (AIDS), first recognized as a disease in June 1981, is the result of infection by a retrovirus known as human immunodeficiency virus (HIV). Three groups of infected patients can be identified:

1. Apparently healthy persons who test positive for antibodies specific to the virus. These antibodies appear within 2–6 months after exposure but are not capable of eradicating the disease. So far only 3% of infected individuals manifest or have died from the full-blown syndrome. Owing to the long incubation period of AIDS infection (6 months to 7 years), it is impossible to say how many of the asymptomatic patients will eventually succumb to the disease.

2. A small group of patients who have a mononucleosis-like infection associated with lymphadenopathy, malaise, unexplained fever, night sweats, diarrhea, and weight loss. If these symptoms persist more than 3 months without resolution or progression to AIDS, the patient is said to have AIDS-related complex (ARC) or persistent lymphadenopathy syndrome (PLS).

3. Patients who have the full-blown syndrome characterized by damage to the immune system due to destruction of T4 (helper) lymphocytes and are predisposed to opportunisitc infections and certain malignancies (*Pneumocystis carinii* pneumonia, cytomegalic and Epstein-Barr virus, herpes simplex; Kaposi's sarcoma, Burkitt's and non-Hodgkin's lymphoma). Neurological manifestations, also common among victims of AIDS, are due to infection of the central nervous system by the virus itself or to malignancies (e.g., lymphoma) and other infections (e.g., toxoplasmosis) involving the central nervous system.

The screening test for HIV infection is a check for specific antibodies by the enzyme-linked immunosorbent assay (ELISA).

Once the serum is found to be positive or reactive it is subjected to a second test for confirmation: either the Western blot test or the immunofluorescent assay (IFA). These last two methods are less sensitive than ELISA but more specific.

EPIDEMIOLOGY OF AIDS

The interval in which the number of reported HIV infections doubles has increased from every 5 months in 1982 to every 13 months in 1988. Therefore the spread of the disease has not been exponential, as was feared earlier. The virus has been isolated largely from genital secretions and blood, and only in small amounts from tears, saliva, feces, and breast milk. Its principal modes of transmission are sexual intercourse and sharing of contaminated hypodermic needles. Sixty-six percent of afflicted patients are homosexual or bisexual men, 17% are intravenous drug users, another 8% are male homosexuals who also abuse drugs, 3% are recipients of contaminated blood products, and 2% are heterosexual partners of persons at high-risk. The virus can cross the placenta from mother to fetus. It is estimated that 35–60% of infants born of infected mothers will acquire the infection.

Although the pattern of AIDS transmission is similar to that of hepatitis B virus infections, the former is considerably less virulent. No reported cases of infection through contact with tears or saliva has occurred, nor has there been report of infection through food, drinks, air, or contact with environmental surfaces. Four tenths of 1% (0.4%) of health care personnel who have open wounds exposed to contaminated blood have developed antibodies to the virus; 75% of these contacts were accidental needle injuries. Similar exposure to blood contaminated with hepatitis B virus would result in a 26% rate of infection.

IMPLICATIONS IN ANESTHETIC PRACTICE

Largely owing to ignorance of the disease, AIDS has struck fear and terror into all segments of society, including physicians. Anesthesiologists are often questioned by patients who are concerned about contracting the disease through blood transfusion, and they will certainly be called to anesthetize AIDS patients or to participate in their treatment sometime in their career. About 5% of all patients seen in the emergency departments of urban hospitals in the United States are seropositive for HIV infection. Therefore the anesthesiologist should be familiar with the current status of the disease and with procedures to contain its spread.

Blood Tranfusion and AIDS

Currently all blood banks have instituted procedures to eliminate blood products as a source of infection by:

1. Encouraging persons from high-risk groups to refrain from donating blood

2. Using the enzyme-linked immunosorbent assay as a screening test and the Western blot or immunofluorescent assay as a confirmatory test for HIV antibodies on all donated blood

3. Subjecting all factor VIII and IX preparations to heat treatment to kill any AIDS virus that may be present.

Because of the latency of 2–6 months between exposure and appearance of antibodies, it is conceivable that an occasional unit of contaminated blood will escape detection. It is estimated that the chances of a surgical patient's contracting the disease following a single unit transfusion are 1 in 40,000. This risk will decrease, or even disappear, when testing for the presence of the HIV antigen in donated blood becomes routine.

Since bank blood is a potential medium for transmission of AIDS and other infectious diseases, the anesthesiologist can help to reduce the incidence of transfusion-related infections by:

1. Choosing techniques that limit blood loss in certain types of surgery (e.g., epidural or spinal anesthesia in pelvic and hip surgery and controlled hypotension in radical cancer surgery)

2. Prescribing blood products judiciously in the perioperative period

3. Using autologous blood or autotransfusion techniques to decrease dependence on bank blood. (Details of the last two topics are found in Chap. 21.)

PRECAUTIONS WHEN TREATING AIDS PATIENTS

Strict isolation techniques should be practiced by health care personnel treating AIDS patients in order to protect patients from seemingly trivial infections (e.g., the common cold) and to avoid contracting the AIDS virus from them. Universal precautions are now advocated in North America: that is, all patients should be treated as potential carriers of the disease. In general precautions practiced for hepatitis B infection also apply to AIDS. Personnel with open wounds, exudative lesions, or weeping dermatitis that cannot be covered effectively should refrain from performing or assisting in procedures in which splashing of blood or body fluid is likely.

General Conduct

Anesthesia personnel should wear waterproof gown, gloves, mask, and goggles when attending AIDS patients. Clean and contaminated areas should be strictly defined on the work table; the contaminated area is best confined to a tray or kidney dish. Since the anesthesiologist must turn to adjusting controls on the anesthetic machine and ventilator immediately following laryngoscopy and intubation, he should be double-gloved for this and similar procedures and should remove the contaminated outer gloves after the procedure before touching clean areas. Household bleach (sodium hypochlorite) diluted in 1–9 parts water is the recommended disinfectant for environmental surfaces. For maximum effectiveness, these surfaces should be washed and let dry for 20 minutes. Other effective disinfectants include 40% ethyl alcohol, 30% isopropyl alcohol, 5% phenol, 2% formalin, 1% Lysol, and 0.1% glutaraldehyde.

Resuscitaton and Anesthetic Equipment

In order to avoid mouth-to-mouth contact during basic life support, a disposable mouthpiece and resuscitation bag (e.g., Brooke's airway and Resuscibag) should be available at the patient's bedside, and health care personnel should be trained in their use. Whenever possible, disposable anesthetic equipment should be employed. Conventional bacterial filters do not protect the anesthetic machine and ventilator from contamination.

Needles and Syringes

Accidental injury by contaminated needle represents the greatest hazard to anesthesia personnel, yet multiple and repeated injections of drugs from one syringe into an indwelling intravenous infusion during the course of the anesthetic are common practice. Modifications are necessary to reduce this hazard:

1. Use only disposable needles and plastic syringes. Use a fresh needle and syringe every time when dispensing drugs from a multidose vial. Never recap needles, even those that are judged clean.

2. Do not use a needle to inject into an infusion line via its injection port. Incorporate a two-way stopcock into the infusion line using an extension set, and inject drugs into the infusion via the stopcock without a needle.

3. Avoid the habit of "piggy-back" using a needle. Remove the rubber bung at the injection port of the main infusion line and connect the distal end of the secondary infusion directly to the injection port.

4. Collect used needles, syringes, and other sharp objects into

a nearby puncture-resistant container labelled "BIOHAZARD." Such materials must be autoclaved before being discarded.

Blood and Fluid Specimens

Blood samples from infected patients should be collected directly into a pre-evacuated specimen tube using the Vacutainer system; they should *not* be collected separately using needle and syringe and then transferred to the specimen tube by puncturing its rubber cap with the contaminated needle. All blood and body fluid specimens should bear the label "BLOOD AND BODY FLUID PRECAUTIONS" and should be sent to the laboratory in a crush-resistant container.

Dealing with Accidents

It is hoped that proper precautions will eliminate all instances of accidential injury by contaminated needles and spattering of blood or body fluid into eyes or mouth. In case of mishaps the following routines are recommended:

1. When blood is splashed onto intact skin, just wash it off with soap and water.
2. When eyes are contaminated, rinse them thoroughly under a running tap.
3. When blood or other fluid gets into the mouth, spit it out and gargle with water or a mouth rinse.
4. When open injury has occurred, press the wound to make it bleed and then wash the affected area with soap and water. Consider active and passive immunization against hepatitis B infection because many AIDS patients are also carriers of that virus.
5. Obtain permission to test the patient serologically if HIV antibody status is unknown.

In all instances other than item 1, the accident should be reported to the Employee Health Department of the institution and the affected person should join a surveillance program for personnel who may have been exposed to the AIDS virus at work. This involves follow-up by serological testing every 4 months for at least 1 year and is designed to determine the risk to health care personnel following accidental exposure to the virus.

Further Reading

AIDS

Lifson AR, Castro KG, McCray E, Jaffe, HW: National surveillance of AIDS in health care workers. JAMA 256:3231, 1986.

Ruthanne M, et al: Surveillance of health care workers exposed to blood from patients infected with the human immunodeficiency virus. N Engl J Med 319:1118, 1988.

Understanding AIDS: Information for Hospitals and Health Professionals. Ottawa, Ontario Ministry of Health, 1988.

Zuck TF: Transfusion-transmitted AIDS reassessed. N Engl J Med 318:511, 1988.

Anesthesia Equipment

Dorsch JA, Dorsch SE: Understanding Anesthesia Equipment, ed 2. St. Louis, CV Mosby, 1984.

Dupuis YG: Ventilators: Theory and Clinical Application. St. Louis, CV Mosby, 1986.

Petty C: The Anesthesia Machine. New York, Churchill-Livingstone, 1987.

History of Anesthesia

Keys TE: The History of Surgical Anesthesia. New York, Schuman, 1945.

Sykes WS: Essays on the First Hundred Years of Anaesthesia, vols I, II and III. Edinburgh, Churchill-Livingstone, 1982.

Malignant Hyperthermia

Symposium on malignant hyperthermia. Br J Anaesth 60:251, 1988.

Mechanisms of Drug Action

Allison AC, Nunn JF: Effects of general anaesthetics on microtubules. Lancet 2:1326, 1968.

Chang KJ, Cooper BR, Hazum E, Cuatrecasas P: Multiple opiate receptors: Different regional distribution in the brain and differential binding of opiates and opioid peptides. Molec Pharmacol 16:91, 1979.

Fink BR: Molecular Mechanisms of Anesthesia. New York, Raven Press, 1975.

Larrabee MG, Posternak JM: Selective action of anesthetics on synapses and axons in mammalian sympathetic ganglia. J Neurophysiol 15:91, 1952.

Millar SL: A theory of gaseous anesthetics. Proc Natl Acad Sci (USA) 47:1515, 1961.

Miller RJ, Cuatrecasas P: Neurobiology and neuropharmacology of the enkephalins. Adv Biochem Psychopharmacol 20:187, 1979.

Pauling L: A molecular theory of general anesthesia. Science 134:15,1961.

Richards CD, Russell WJ, Smaje JC: The action of ether and methoxyflurane on synaptic transmission in isolated preparations of the mammalian cortex. J Physiol (Lond) 248:121, 1975.

Roth SH, Miller KW: Cellular and Molecular Mechanisms of Anesthetics. New York, Plenum Press, 1986.

Saubermann AJ, Gallagher ML: Mechanisms of general anesthesia: Failure of pentobarbital and halothane to depolymerize microtubules in mouse optic nerve. Anesthesiology 38:25, 1973.

Seeman P: The membrane actions of anesthetics and tranquillizers. Pharmacol Rev 24:583, 1972.

Strichartz G: Molecular mechanisms of nerve block by local anesthetics. Anesthesiology 45:421, 1976.

Trudell JR: A unitary theory of anesthesia based on lateral phase separations in nerve membrane. Anesthesiology 46:5, 1977.

Monitoring

Gravenstein JS, Paulus DA: Clinical Monitoring Practice, ed 2. Philadelphia, JB Lippincott, 1987.

Lam AM: Monitoring evoked neurologic responses. American Society of Anesthesiologists Refresher Course 155:1, 1988.

Lubbers DW: Theoretical basis of the transcutaneous blood gas measurements. Crit Care Med 9:721, 1981.

Merilainen PT: Metabolic monitor. Int J Clin Monit Comput 4:167, 1987.

Ozanne JW, Young WG, Mazzei WJ, Severinghaus JW: Multipatient anesthetic mass spectrometry: Rapid analysis of data stored in long catheters. Anesthesiology 55:62, 1981.

Swedlow DB: Capnometry and capnography: An anesthesia disaster warning system. Semin Anesthesia 5:194, 1986.

VanWagenen RA, Westenskow DR, Benner RE, Gregonis DE, Coleman DL: Dedicated monitoring of anesthetic and respiratory gases by Raman scattering. J Clin Monit 2:215, 1986.

Yelderman M, New W: Evaluation of pulse oximetry. Anesthesiology 59:349, 1983.

Quality Assurance and Risk Management

Adams AK: Quality assurance in anaesthesia. Anaesthesia 38:311, 1983.

Cooper JB, Newbower RS, Kitz RJ: An analysis of major errors and equipment failures in anesthesia management: Considerations for prevention and detection. Anesthesiology 60:34, 1984.

Council on Medical Service: Guidelines for quality assurance. JAMA 259:2572, 1988.

Davies JM, Strunin L: Anesthesia in 1984: How safe is it? Can Med Assoc J 131:437, 1984.

Duberman SM: Quality Assurance in the Practice of Anesthesiology. American Society of Anesthesiologists, 1986.

Resuscitation

American Medical Association: Standards and guidelines for cardiopulmonary resuscitation and emergency cardiac care. Part II: Adult basic life support. JAMA 255:2915, 1986.

American Medical Association: Standards and guidelines for cardiopulmonary resuscitation and emergency cardiac care. Part III: Adult advanced cardiac life support. JAMA 255:2933, 1986.

American Medical Association: Standards and guidelines for cardiopulmonary resuscitation and emergency cardiac care. Part IV: Pediatric basic life support. JAMA 255:2954, 1986.

American Medical Association: Standards and guidelines for cardiopulmonary resuscitation and emergency cardiac care. Part V: Pediatric advanced life support. JAMA 255:2961, 1986.

American Medical Association: Standards and guidelines for cardiopulmonary resuscitation and emergency cardiac care. Part VI: Neonatal advanced life support. JAMA 255:2969, 1986.

American Medical Association: Standards and guidelines for cardiopulmonary resuscitation and emergency cardiac care. Part VIII: Medicolegal considerations and recommendations. JAMA 255:2979, 1986.

Transfusion

American Medical Association Council Report: Autologous blood transfusion. JAMA 256:2378, 1986.

Blood Transfusion Therapy: A Physician's Handbook, ed 4. Arlington, VA, American Association of Blood Banks, 1987.

Clinical Guide to Transfusion: Products and Practices. Ottawa, The Canadian Red Cross Society Blood Services, 1987.

Specialty Textbooks

Albright GA, Ferguson JE III, Stevenson DK, Joyce TH III: Anesthesia in Obstetrics: Maternal, Fetal, and Neonatal Aspects, ed 2. London, Butterworths, 1986.

Benumof JL: Anesthesia for Thoracic Surgery. Philadelphia, WB Saunderes, 1987.

Cousins MJ, Bridenbaugh PO: Neural Blockade. Philadelphia, JB Lippincott, 1988.

Ellis H, Feldman S: Anatomy for Anaesthetists. London, Blackwell, 1988.

Fragen RJ: New Anesthetic Drugs. Philadelphia, WB Saunders, 1988.

Goudsouzian N, Karamanian A: Physiology for the Anesthesiologist, ed 2. Norwalk, CT, Appleton & Lange, 1984.

Gregory GA: Pediatric Anesthesia. New York, Churchill-Livingstone, 1983.

Lake CL: Cardiovascular Anesthesia. Berlin, Springer-Verlag, 1985.

Lubin MF, Walker HK, Smith RB III: Medical Management of the Surgical Patient, ed 2. London, Butterworths, 1987.

Martin JT: Positioning in Anesthesia and Surgery, ed 2. Philadelphia, WB Saunders, 1988.

Newfield P, Cottrell JE: Handbook of Neuroanesthesia: Clinical and Physiologic Essentials. Boston, Little, Brown, 1983.

Nunn JF: Applied Respiratory Physiology, ed 3. London, Butterworths, 1987.

Patil VU, Stehling LC, Zauder HL: Fiberoptic Endoscopy in Anesthesia. Chicago, Year Book, 1983.

Stephen CR, Assaf RAE: Geriatric Anesthesia. London, Butterworths, 1986.

Stoelting RK: Pharmacology and Physiology in Anesthetic Practice. Philadelphia, JB Lippincott, 1987.

Stoelting RK, Dierdorf SF, McCammon RL: Anesthesia and Co-existing Disease, ed 2. New York, Churchill-Livingstone, 1988.

Swerdlow M: Relief of Intractable Pain, ed 3. Amsterdam, Elsevier, 1983.

Wetchler BV: Anesthesia for Ambulatory Surgery. Philadelphia, JB Lippincott, 1985.

Anesthesia Journals

Anaesthesia, Academic Press.
Anaesthesia and Intensive Care, Australian Society of Anaesthetists.
Anesthesia and Analgesia, Elsevier.
Anesthesiology, JB Lippincott.
British Journal of Anaesthesia, MacMillan.
Canadian Journal of Anaesthesia, Canadian Anaesthetists' Society.
The Clinical Journal of Pain, Raven Press.
European Journal of Anaesthesiology, Blackwell.
Journal of Cardiothoracic Anesthesia, Grune & Stratton.
Journal of Neurosurgical Anesthesiology, Raven Press.
Regional Anesthesia, JB Lippincott.

American Society of Anesthesiologists: Standards for Basic Intraoperative Monitoring*

These standards apply to all anesthesia care, although in emergency circumstances appropriate life support measures take precedence. These standards may be exceeded at any time based on the judgment of the responsible anesthesiologist. They are intended to encourage high quality patient care, but observing them cannot guarantee any specific patient outcome. They are subject to revision from time to time, as warranted by the evolution of technology and practice. This set of standards addresses only the issue of basic intraoperative monitoring, which is one component of anesthesia care. In certain rare or unusual circumstances, (1) some of these methods of monitoring may be clinically impractical, and (2) appropriate use of the described monitoring methods may fail to detect untoward clinical developments. Brief interruptions of continual monitoring may be unavoidable. Under extenuating circumstances, the responsible anesthesiologist may waive the requirements marked with an asterisk (*); it is recommended that when this is done, it should be so stated (including the reasons) in a note in the patient's medical record. These standards are not intended for application to the care of the obstetrical patient in labor or in the conduct of pain management.

(Note that "continual" is defined as "repeated regularly and frequently in steady succession" whereas "continuous" means "prolonged without any interruption at any time.")

---

* Reproduced with the permission of the American Society of Anesthesiologists.

STANDARD I

Qualified anesthesia personnel shall be present in the room throughout the conduct of all general anesthetics, regional anesthetics, and monitored anesthesia care.

Objective:

Because of the rapid changes in patient status during anesthesia, qualified anesthesia personnel shall be continuously present to monitor the patient and provide anesthesia care. In the event there is a direct known hazard, e.g., radiation to the anesthesia personnel, which might require intermittent remote observation of the patient, some provision for monitoring the patient must be made. In the event that an emergency requires the temporary absence of the person primarily responsible for the anesthetic, the best judgment of the anesthesiologist will be exercised in comparing the emergency with the anesthetized patient's condition and in the selection of the person left responsible for the anesthetic during the temporary absence.

STANDARD II

During all anesthetics, the patient's oxygenation, ventilation, circulation, and temperature shall be continually evaluated.

Oxygenation

Objective:

To ensure adequate oxygen concentration in the inspired gas and the blood during all anesthetics.

Methods:

(1) Inspired gas. During every administration of general anesthesia using an anesthesia machine, the concentration of oxygen in the patient breathing system shall be measured by an oxygen analyzer with a low oxygen concentration limit alarm in use.

(2) Blood oxygenation. During all anesthetics, a quantitative method of assessing oxygenation such as pulse oximetry shall be employed. Adequate illumination and exposure of the patient is necessary to assess color.

Ventilation

Objective:

To ensure adequate ventilation of the patient during all anesthetics.

Methods:

(1) Every patient receiving general anesthesia shall have the adequacy of ventilation continually evaluated. While qualitative clinical signs such as chest excursion, observation of the reservoir breathing bag, and auscultation of breath sounds may be adequate, quantitative monitoring of the CO_2 content and/or volume of gas is encouraged.

(2) When an endotracheal tube is inserted, its correct positioning in the trachea must be verified. Clinical assessment is essential and end-tidal CO_2 analysis, in use from the time of endotracheal tube placement, is encouraged.

(3) When ventilation is controlled by a mechanical ventilator, there shall be in continuous use a device that is capable of detecting disconnection of components of the breathing system. The device must give an audible signal when its alarm threshold is exceeded.

(4) During regional anesthesia and monitored anesthesia care, the adequacy of ventilation shall be evaluated, at least, by continual observation of qualitative clinical signs.

Circulation

Objective:

To ensure the adequacy of the patient's circulatory function during all anesthetics.

Methods:

(1) Every patient receiving anesthesia shall have the electrocardiogram continuously displayed from the beginning of anesthesia until preparing to leave the anesthetizing location.

(2) Every patient receiving anesthesia shall have arterial blood pressure and heart rate determined and evaluated at least every 5 minutes.

(3) Every patient receiving general anesthesia shall have, in addition to the above, circulatory function continually evaluated by at least one of the following: palpation of a pulse, auscultation of heart sounds, monitoring of a tracing of intra-arterial pressure, ultrasound peripheral pulse monitoring, or pulse plethysmography or oximetry.

Body Temperature

Objective:

To aid in the maintenance of appropriate body temperature during all anesthetics.

Methods:

There shall be readily available a means to continuously measure the patient's temperature. When changes in body temperature are intended, anticipated, or suspected, the temperature shall be measured.

Dosages of Commonly Used Anesthetic Drugs*

	INDUCTION OR INITIAL DOSE	MAINTENANCE DOSE
INTRAVENOUS AGENTS		
Thiopental	3–5 mg/kg	
Methohexital	1–2 mg/kg	
Diazepam	0.15–1.5 mg/kg	
Midazolam	0.15–0.4 mg/kg	
Ketamine	1–2 mg/kg IV	
	6.5–13 mg/kg IM	
Etomidate	0.25–0.3 mg/kg	
Propofol	1.5–3.0 mg/kg	
INHALATION AGENTS		
Nitrous oxide		50–70%
Halothane	Up to 4%	0.5–1.5%
Enflurane	Up to 5%	0.5–3.0%
Isoflurane	Up to 5%	0.5–2.5%
NARCOTIC ANALGESICS		
Morphine[†]	5–10 mg	1–2 mg prn
Meperidine	50–100 mg	10–20 mg prn
Fentanyl[†]	1.0–3.0 µg/kg	10–25 µg prn
Sufentanil[†]	0.2–0.7 µg/kg	5–10 µg prn
Alfentanil	By titration	Not to exceed 5–40 µg/kg in 30 min or 75 µg/kg in 1 hour
	50–75 µg/kg	0.5–1.5 µg/kg/min for operations longer than 1 hour

	INDUCTION OR INITIAL DOSE	MAINTENANCE DOSE
NARCOTIC ANTAGONISTS		
Naloxone	1.0–1.5 µg/kg	
MUSCLE RELAXANTS		
Succinylcholine	1 mg/kg	
d-Tubocurarine	0.3–0.4 mg/kg	0.1 mg/kg prn
Pancuronium	0.06–0.08 mg/kg	0.01–0.02 mg/kg prn
Metocurine	0.15–0.2 mg/kg	0.03 mg/kg prn
Gallamine	1.5–2.0 mg/kg	0.5 mg/kg prn
Atracurium	0.3–0.4 mg/kg	0.08–0.1 mg/kg prn
Vecuronium	0.08–1.0 mg/kg	0.01–0.02 mg/kg prn
MUSCLE RELAXANT ANTAGONISTS[‡]		
Neostigmine	0.03–0.07 mg/kg	
Pyridostigmine	0.15–0.3 mg/kg	
Edrophonium	0.5–1.0 mg/kg	

* All doses are recommended as guidelines only. Actual dose must be titrated to the patient's response, with consideration of concurrent medications, patient's condition, and surgical procedure. All doses are given IV unless otherwise specified.

[†] Doses recommended are for supplemental analgesia only. Doses are increased 10- to 30-fold when used as primary anesthetic agents.

[‡] Muscle relaxant antagonists must be given with a vagolytic agent to prevent muscarinic side-effects.

Index

Note: Page numbers in *italics* refer to illustrations; page numbers followed by t refer to tables.